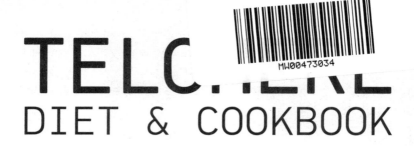

TELOMERE
DIET & COOKBOOK

A cutting-edge holistic guide to living younger longer! You'll savor the doable and delicious recipes and menus designed with your telomeres in mind for the healthiest life possible.

—Kathie Madonna Swift, MS, RDN, Food as Medicine program director, Center for Mind-Body Medicine

The Telomere Diet and Cookbook offers a new angle for applying the science of healthy eating and living. Maggie Moon provides nourishing whole-food recipes to promote healthy aging and protect our DNA. While the concept is relatively new, this book offers cutting-edge information and practical recommendations for staying ahead of the curve.

—Kelly Morrow, MS, RDN, FAND, Bastyr University and the Bastyr Center for Natural Health

Maggie Moon takes the emerging and somewhat complex topic of telomeres and provides easy-to-understand information as well as practical and delectable ideas about how to put them into play. For anyone interested in scientifically sound—yet forward-thinking and holistic—approaches to aging, this innovative guide may be like having the fountain of youth on your bookshelf!

—Mary Purdy, MS, RDN, speaker, author, functional nutrition practitioner, and past chair of Dietitians in Integrative and Functional Medicine

Maggie Moon helps us improve our health span by explaining the emerging science on telomeres and aging in her latest book, *The Telomere Diet and Cookbook*. Her unique plant-forward diet plan and delicious recipes will help put you on the path to optimal aging.

—Christine Rosenbloom, PhD, RDN, FAND, author of *Food & Fitness After 50*

The intersection of telomeres and nutrition is fascinating and complicated. Dietitian author Moon expertly navigates this subject in a relatable way and provides absolutely delicious recipes along the way.

—Ginger Hultin, MS, RDN, CSO, owner of the concierge nutrition practice Champagne Nutrition

The Telomere Diet and Cookbook provides an excellent primer on an emerging scientific area of study on how our diet and lifestyle choices can impact our longevity. Maggie Moon, renowned registered dietitian, breaks down complex science into understandable terms and offers simple advice along with delicious recipes for keeping our telomeres healthy.

—Linda Cornish, founder and president, Seafood Nutrition Partnership

TELOMERE
DIET & COOKBOOK

A Scientific Approach to Slow Your Genetic
Aging and Live a Longer, Healthier Life

MAGGIE MOON, MS, RD

Published in the United States by:
Ulysses Press
P.O. Box 3440
Berkeley, CA 94703
www.ulyssespress.com

ISBN: 978-1-61243-929-7
Library of Congress Catalog Number: 2019905615

Printed in Canada by Marquis Book Printing
10 9 8 7 6 5 4 3 2 1

Acquisitions editor: Casie Vogel
Managing editor: Claire Chun
Editor: Susan Lang
Proofreader: Kate St. Clair
Cover design: David Hastings
Layout: Jake Flaherty

IMPORTANT NOTE TO READERS: This book has been written and published for informational and educational purposes only. It is not intended to serve as medical advice or to be any form of medical treatment. You should always consult with your physician before altering or changing any aspect of your medical treatment. Do not stop or change any prescription medications without the guidance and advice of your physician. Any use of the information in this book is made on the reader's good judgment and is the reader's sole responsibility. This book is not intended to diagnose or treat any medical condition and is not a substitute for a physician. This book is independently authored and published and no sponsorship or endorsement of this book by, and no affiliation with, any trademarked brands or other products mentioned within is claimed or suggested. All trademarks that appear in ingredient lists and elsewhere in this book belong to their respective owners and are used here for informational purposes only. The author and publisher encourage readers to patronize the quality brands mentioned in this book.

For Fred, the one I want to grow old with.

CONTENTS

Chapter 5

RECIPES 120

INTRODUCTION

The Telomere Diet and Cookbook is a practical, evidence-based guide to living more years in good health, by way of the kitchen. The exciting discovery of how the telomeres in every single one of our cells work reveals a new way to understand the systemic whole-body process of aging. The latest science on telomeres exposes how the way we eat, sleep, respond to stress, and interact with others may impact how we age: everyday habits can accelerate or slow down aging.

As life expectancies rise worldwide, it has become apparent that while some people thrive as they age, many others spend years unduly burdened by preventable chronic disease. Think of someone you know who is your same chronological age but whose vitality is more like someone much younger or older than you. This is the difference between health span and life span. While aging is complicated, telomeres offer a new window into understanding it. Research suggests those with healthier telomeres live longer and in better health.

In 2009, the Nobel Prize in Physiology or Medicine was awarded to a team of scientists for uncovering how telomeres and the enzyme telomerase protect chromosomes. The scientific community has continued to study and learn more about telomeres ever since. This book explains the best available science on the intersection of telomeres, nutrition, and health in understandable terms. Then it puts that exciting emerging research in the larger context of established credible nutrition science. The result is a plant-based, but not plant-exclusive, eating pattern based on a variety of wholesome foods such as vegetables, fruit, nuts, beans, seafood, whole grains, tea, and more.

Most importantly, this book provides practical tips and tools to apply the research findings to your everyday life. To bring it all together, the book offers a simple step-by-step starter program for your best telomere health. The program is holistic in its lifestyle approach. It provides detailed meal plans and shopping lists, including when it's OK to seek out supplements, as well as specific guidance on exercise, stress reduction, and healthy sleep.

All the great-tasting, inflammation-busting, antioxidant-rich recipes you need to get started are included. The book features recipes for breakfasts, entrées, snacks, sides, desserts, and drinks. You'll find familiar comfort foods with a healthy twist, so there's no need to give up your favorite flavors. You'll also find dishes inspired by global cuisines and healthy eating trends that bring modern variety to your table. Thankfully, on-trend does not mean fussy: the recipes have the home cook in mind and are designed to maximize flavor and minimize effort. Developed by yours truly, a culinary school–trained registered dietitian, the recipes offer the best of both worlds: they were made to taste great and are nutritionist approved!

My goal is to get you eating wholesome foods for telomere health as quickly and effectively as possible. But I also want you to understand and easily find the science behind the recommendations on specific nutrients, foods, and eating patterns. Therefore, the book is organized for you to skip right to an action plan, but also makes it easy to find the science.

It's important to me that you understand how young this science is. We still have a lot to learn in this exciting corner of the scientific world, but I'm excited to share what we know so far about telomeres and healthy lifestyles. This is my perspective: if there's little to no risk, potential telomere benefit, and likely other benefit to eating certain foods and engaging in certain lifestyle habits, then I want you to know about it and give you practical ideas to make it part of your life.

I truly hope this book helps you make healthy choices, feel great, and live well.

In good health,
Maggie Moon

CHAPTER 1

THE BASICS

Before we dive into what telomeres are from a technical perspective, let me tell you why they are important. Telomeres are a marker for aging, much in the same way that cholesterol is a marker for heart health. Similarly, diet and lifestyle can have a positive or negative effect on telomeres. This chapter will provide basic background information on how telomeres were discovered, what they are, what they do, and how they work.

A BRIEF HISTORY
OF TELOMERE SCIENCE

When it comes to what we know about telomeres and health, the science has had a few pivotal moments, with many more surely to come. Anyone interested in telomeres should know about these milestones:

• In 1962, Leonard Hayflick developed the "Hayflick limit," a telomere-based theory that says human life span can reach a maximum of 120 years, because this is the time it takes for the telomeres of enough cells to be so eroded and shortened that the cells stop dividing and replicating.

- In 1971, Alexey Olovnikov hypothesized that a little bit of DNA was lost every time cells divided and chromosomes replicated.

- In the early 2000s, Elizabeth Blackburn published data suggesting that the enzyme telomerase could repair very short or dysfunctional telomeres.

- In 2009, Drs. Blackburn, Greider, and Szostak received the Nobel Prize in Physiology or Medicine for the discovery of how telomeres and telomerase work to protect chromosomes. What they learned about telomerase opened the door to a way around the Hayflick limit.

- In 2019, the term "telomere" appeared in more than 22,000 academic papers indexed in the U.S. National Library of Medicine's PubMed database.

TELOMERES: WHAT THEY ARE AND HOW THEY WORK

Telomeres, bits of expendable noncoding DNA that sit at the ends of chromosomes, are a relatively new biomarker for aging. They dwindle naturally over time as a part of normal aging. Every time a cell divides, telomeres get a little shorter. This is normal. Cells can also be triggered to divide as a reaction to inflammation and oxidative stress, leading to premature telomere shortening. This premature and accelerated dwindling can be caused by a poor diet, sedentary lifestyle, chronic illness, or infection. Think of telomeres as a new way to measure biological aging on a cellular level, similar to the way cholesterol and blood pressure are used as markers for overall heart health.

As I mentioned, telomeres sit at the ends of chromosomes, which are full of DNA code. They are often compared to the plastic tips of shoelaces, without which the laces (chromosomes, in this analogy) would fray, come undone, and fail to work the right way. Telomeres protect the strands of DNA in chromosomes from damage. This is important because our chromosomes carry the genetic code that makes us uniquely who we are. When cells divide and new cells replace old ones, healthy chromosomes with ample telomeres shed some length but not enough to damage the coding DNA. Therefore, the DNA that makes us who we are remains intact. This is why protecting telomeres is essential.

WHY DO CELLS DIVIDE?

Cells divide so that they can multiply, making new cells for the body to use. Different organs have different rates of turnover. For example, tens of thousands of skin cells are replaced each day (with 100% turnover in about a month), while only about 700 neurons in the brain's hippocampus do the same (that's an annual turnover of about 1.75%). This kind of cell division is called mitosis, and it's fundamental to life.

During mitosis a cell duplicates itself and divides into two identical cells. The process is tightly regulated and has quality assurance checkpoints at which certain genes can stop the cycle for repairs as needed. If a cell's DNA error is irreparable, it may be cleared away through a process called apoptosis, also known as programmed cell death. Apoptosis is the body's inherent mechanism to clear away damaged cells that could otherwise lead to cancer.

Only a few cells hold on to long telomeres: egg, sperm, and cancer cells. Most cells have telomeres that naturally diminish over time.

While we don't want telomeres that dwindle too quickly, it's important to understand that healthy telomeres don't live forever, either. Most cells go through a natural life cycle ending in death and clearance (see Why Do Cells Divide? above). The natural life cycle of a cell, along with gradual telomere shortening, is in place to protect against cancerous tumors, which are full of cells that never want to die. Healthy telomeres prevent chromosomes from rearranging themselves abnormally, potentially leading to immortal cancer cells. Telomeres also work by keeping chromosome ends from fusing and sticking to each other, which impacts their stability. Such dysfunctional telomeres are associated with late-life diseases such as Parkinson's disease, Alzheimer's disease, heart disease, and cancer.

There are rare genetic conditions, called telomere syndromes, in which telomeres don't work well. People with telomere syndromes, even children with these conditions, age prematurely and show signs and symptoms more common to geriatric patients. However, most cases of prematurely shrinking telomeres are related to nongenetic (aka lifestyle) factors.

TECHNICALLY SPEAKING

Telomeres are strips of noncoding DNA called nucleotides, which sit on the ends of each and every one of our chromosomes. They are made of simple and disposable DNA sequences that do not contain any of our genetic code. They act as protective buffers against chromosome damage by taking the brunt of cell division so the chromosome and its genetic code remain safe. If chromosomes were quarterbacks, telomeres would be the offensive line. They look like this: 5'-TTAGGG-3' and 3'-CCCTAA-5'.

HOW LONG SHOULD MY TELOMERES BE?

Unfortunately, the answer is neither brief nor straightforward.

One, women tend to have longer telomeres than men, although the exact reasons are unknown. However, several population-wide studies confirm the finding. Studies that include both men and women sometimes report different findings for how much good nutrition and exercise impact telomere length, even though there is still a general case to be made for both sexes to engage in these healthy lifestyle factors.

Two, each type of chromosome has a normal range for the length of its telomeres. That varies again by each type of cell (e.g., white blood cells, muscle cells, bone marrow cells). It adds up to thousands and thousands of telomere DNA base-pairs. The length of a person's telomeres is described in comparison with those of an age-matched healthy population, so it is a dynamic measurement that is hard to pin down. Even so, the overall length of telomere DNA is not what's most significant. Just a handful of overly short telomeres can cause DNA damage; therefore, it may be more important to know how many short or long telomeres are within a certain type of cell. Right now, these questions are best asked in research settings, not doctors' offices.

What we do know is that average telomere length is a reliable predictor of health span, or years of life spent in good health, as well as overall longevity. Throughout this book, when we discuss telomere length, it refers to the average telomere length in the body. Emerging evidence suggests that modern lifestyles are causing our telomeres to deteriorate too quickly, but don't let that make you think longer is always better. In fact, you know what type of cells have long telomeres that don't seem to diminish much? Cancer cells. They want to live forever. Both extremes—too short and too long—seem to result in negative health consequences. It's all about balance. And, OK, moderate lengthening might be a good thing, but we'll get to that.

WHAT CAN I DO TO KEEP MY TELOMERES HEALTHY?

We are born with certain length telomeres. We don't have any control over the telomere length we start with. However, daily lifestyle habits of what we eat, how much we move and sleep, and how we handle stress can influence how much oxidative stress and inflammation we expose our telomeres to. Research has shown that healthy diets and lifestyles are associated with telomere health.

If we assume that the gradual loss of telomeres over the years is a marker of normal aging and that certain lifestyle habits accelerate that loss, then the more we learn about what triggers telomere shortening may lead the way to methods for living more years in good health.

WHAT IS TELOMERASE?

Telomerase is an enzyme that adds DNA back to telomeres. It reverses the loss of telomere length.

If chemistry class was a long time ago for you, telomerase may read like a misspelling of telomeres. However, it's a different but related term. Here's a quick tip: molecules ending with "ase" tend to be enzymes. Enzymes mean change. For example, proteases change dietary protein from the foods we eat into smaller amino acids, which the body can use to build other protein structures (fun fact: all enzymes are proteins), hormones, and neurotransmitters. Telomerase is an enzyme that can change our telomeres. It can stabilize and rebuild eroding telomeres, resulting in well-protected chromosomes. Recall that telomeres are long strands of nucleotides at the ends of our chromosomes (like the protective ends of shoelaces). Telomerase adds nucleotides to the ends of each chromosome, effectively reversing the shortening of telomeres that eventually leads to instability and dysfunction.

Telomerase is active in reproductive and stem cells, but at low or undetectable levels in the body's other cells. Even normal stem cells, which do have some active telomerase, don't contain enough to make up for the normal telomere shortening that happens, and so telomeres gradually shorten over time in these cells too.

Telomerase may be both a target to attack in cancers and an agent for lengthening healthy cells' telomeres in the future. This is a current area of study.

HOW ARE TELOMERES MEASURED?

Telomeres are most commonly measured in white blood cells, also called leukocytes. In shorthand, leukocyte telomere length is abbreviated to LTL, and much of the research on diet, lifestyle, and telomeres is by LTL. Leukocytes are easily available to researchers, and it wasn't always clear if LTL was a good measure for telomere length (TL) in other kinds of cells. As recently as 2011, the issue was under debate. However, LTL is now an accepted measure of total body telomere health in all cells except reproductive cells. Research has shown that rates of telomere shortening are similar in leukocytes and other somatic cells (all nonreproductive cells).

IS TELOMERE TESTING READY FOR PRIME TIME?

Experts have mixed opinions on whether a mail-in kit, or even your family doctor, should offer you a telomere test as part of your next routine visit. Yes, there are conditions in which molecular medicine can identify patients who are prone to short- or long-telomere syndrome, which, in turn, can lead to better patient understanding and care. However, there are concerns that we don't yet know enough to reliably interpret test results in most clinical settings and that the usefulness for healthy adults is limited, unless someone has a family history or other signs of a telomere-related disease. On the other hand, some experts think the results could reflect a good measure of a person's overall health and may one day be as common as a cholesterol test. One thing experts do agree on: telomere testing is a valuable medical research tool.

INFLAMMATION

Inflammation and telomere length are closely related, so it's important to provide a brief overview of what it is. Inflammation is a process that occurs in the body's immune system to fight infection, foreign or domestic. The body's white blood cells create chemicals to protect the body from bacterial and viral infections (foreign invaders) as well as autoimmune reactions (domestic attacks, aka fighting our own body's normal cells) in conditions such as allergies and many types of arthritis. These chemicals increase blood flow to the infection area, which leads to redness and warmth, and swelling if fluid leaks as a part of this process. This, in turn, can trigger nerves that sense pain. When more and more inflammatory chemicals gather, they can cause joint irritation and swelling, even wearing down the cartilage that provides a cushion between the ends of bones. Inflammation also creates oxidative stress.

OXIDATIVE STRESS

Oxidative stress describes the imbalance between DNA-damaging free radicals and the body's ability to neutralize them through antioxidants. While the body creates some of its own antioxidants, it does not produce enough to manage the oxidative load coming from environmental factors such as poor diet, pollution, radiation (including sun exposure), and smoking, as well as the normal production of some free radicals from everyday processes such as eating and exercising.

We are more susceptible to oxidative stress as we get older because the body's internal antioxidant production system becomes less efficient. That makes it even more important to increase our intake of antioxidants from dietary sources. In particular, the heart and brain are sensitive to oxidative stress because they are exposed to quite a bit of oxygen and their cells renew more slowly than others. The good news is that higher intakes of antioxidants from food can reduce oxidative stress, improve the immune system, and increase healthy years of life. Eating more antioxidants has been linked to lower risk and better management of diabetes, heart disease, and neurological disorders.

Dietary antioxidants can be vitamins, minerals, or other phytonutrients (plant chemicals), and they come from healthy foods such as fruits, vegetables, seafood, nuts, beans, and spices. By definition, they diminish the negative effects of reactive oxygen species (ROS), reactive nitrogen species (RNS), or both. Many important antioxidants such as vitamin A and zinc also help maintain cell membrane stability. Some of the most important dietary antioxidants are vitamin C, vitamin E, carotenoids (including vitamin A, beta-carotene, lutein, and lycopene), selenium, and zinc. Many plant compounds called polyphenols, such as those found in Concord grape juice, pomegranate juice, green tea, and more, are also being studied for their antioxidant properties. Antioxidant-rich foods include berries, citrus fruit, dark leafy green vegetables, carrots, broccoli, sweet potatoes, tomatoes, olive oil, fish, nuts, tea, spices, garlic, and onion.

RESEARCH IN CONTEXT

The science of telomeres is still relatively young. Telomere length is considered a novel but increasingly accepted measure of biological aging. Some studies report mixed results. Rather than cherry-pick positive results, I will be sharing positive, negative, and neutral results. This can be frustrating at times, when the answer isn't clear, but sometimes that's the truth: the answer isn't clear. In the meantime, it's important to be transparent that we are still learning so much about telomere health and to watch this space for future developments.

Some studies have found no relationship between telomeres and disease, although there were findings for health span. One study of more than 3,000 men and women 70 to 79 years old found that longer telomere length measured in older adults was not related to survival or risk of death from infectious diseases, cancer, and heart disease compared to people with shorter telomeres. However, longer telomeres were significantly and positively associated with more years of healthy life. Therefore, the researchers noted that while telomere length may not be a good biomarker for survival in older populations, it may be an informative marker for healthy aging.

In another study, genetically longer telomeres were linked to an increased risk of developing some cancers while reducing the risk for cardiovascular diseases. This study examined inherited telomere length rather than the impact of lifestyle choices on telomeres.

The bottom line: We are still learning what telomere length can tell us about our health. In the meantime, the lifestyle changes that seem to keep our telomeres healthy, as supported by the emerging science on telomeres, are well in line with sound advice from trusted health experts and major medical associations to eat well, stay active, manage stress, sleep soundly, and nurture meaningful relationships with each other. Weighing the risks versus benefits, a lifestyle that may be good for your telomeres is good for a lot of reasons, and the risk is low.

WHAT IS AGING?

Life expectancy is on the rise, and along with it, the number of adults living into their seventies, eighties, and nineties. By 2060, one in four people in the United States will be 65 years or older. Surviving is one thing, but thriving is another. It is the difference between life span and health span. A longer life span brings with it the opportunities to age well, and the challenges of an increased risk of age-related diseases such as cardiovascular disease, cancers, and neurodegenerative diseases. The latter are measured in Disability Adjusted Life Years (DALY).

In the United States, today's adults 65 years and older can expect about 4 to 7 of their remaining 17 to 19 years to be in poor health. Across states, Mississippi is on the poor end of the health spectrum, and Vermont on the healthy end. Across the country, total Healthy Life Expectancy (HLE) ranges from about 75 to 80 years, with some populations outside these ranges. Here's another way to look at it: the percentage of one's life spent in good health ranges from a low of 61.5% of years in Mississippi to a high of 78.2% in Vermont.

Up to 80% of age-related diseases, such as cancer, type 2 diabetes, and heart disease, are fueled by lifestyle choices—primarily diet and physical activity—according to the Centers for Diseases Control and Prevention (CDC) and the World Health Organization (WHO). Lifestyle changes could reduce age-related diseases by 40% to 80%.

CHRONOLOGICAL VS. BIOLOGICAL AGING

Chronological aging is straightforward. It's measured in birthdays and the passage of time. However, biological aging is the concern of this book. Understanding how we age, and what we can do about it will help us live our best lives for as long as possible. This is good news for us and everyone who cares about us. Yes, there are things we can't change—like how long the telomeres we're born with are or a family history of heart disease. But there are plenty of variables that impact our telomeres and the process of aging that we absolutely have a say in. Let's start by understanding a bit more about aging.

We start aging as soon as we're born, but it's more than the simple passage of time. That ticking of time describes chronological aging. Biological aging is seen and felt through changes in our appearance, physical abilities, and cognition over time. The effects of aging do become more common with more years on this planet, but it is highly variable. A 2019 study did a global assessment of the age at which people felt 65, and it ranged from 76 years old in Japan to 46 years old in Papua New Guinea. This is biological aging: the gradual and progressive deterioration of integrity across organs.

A large portion of our planet's population is aging, and if we can help people live biologically younger for more years, we can improve their quality of life and reduce the burden of disease for them and their caregivers. It's never too late to adopt healthy habits, but many of the chronic diseases plaguing older adults have been decades in the making. It's hard to sell young adults on prevention when they look and feel great. However, it might be an easier case to make now that we have research showing that biological aging is measurable in our thirties.

A 2015 study by Belsky and colleagues was able to quantify biological aging in more than 900 younger adults through

18 measures, including telomeres. They followed young adults from ages 26 to 38 and found varying levels of disease markers one to two decades before they'd be diagnosed. The results clearly showed that adults of the same chronological age could be very different biological ages. At age 38, the participants were biologically aged anywhere from their early thirties to nearly 50, with most falling between biological ages of 37 and 40.

Adults who were biologically older showed a faster pace of aging over the 12-year study. Aging was measured by functionality, brain health, self-awareness of physical well-being, and facial appearance. Based on pacing data, the study suggested that half of the differences in aging across the 38-year-olds could be the result of the 12 years between 26 and 38 years of chronological age.

Biologically older adults scored lower on tests of balance, strength, and motor coordination, and mentioned more physical limitations. They scored lower on IQ tests and their blood vessels showed risk factors for stroke and dementia. Their self-reported health status was worse than those who were biologically younger. People who were not familiar with the group were able to identify differences in biologically older and younger adults based on just photographs.

While measuring aging is controversial, doing so could provide a level of awareness in younger adults and prompt them to adopt healthier habits before they develop age-related diseases. Consider people in your own life who may be the same age but may be very different in terms of overall vitality. Even anecdotally, you can probably think of a few examples that support the Belsky study's findings. Researchers often measure signs of aging after age 65, but as the study noted, the process starts much earlier.

WHAT IS SUCCESSFUL AGING?

The best-known definition of successful aging comes from a late 1990s theory called the Rowe and Kahn model. It describes successful aging as the ability to stay free of disease and disability, maintain high cognitive and physical abilities, and be engaged with life. While this is a useful place to start, it oversimplifies what impacts aging.

Recent thinking adds a more dynamic perspective to the model, and describes successful aging as a lifelong process. A comprehensive look at successful aging considers early childhood influences, socioeconomic structures of race, gender, and social class, and the time in history in which we live. This update to the model from other researchers takes a long view of aging, and shows how there is hope for growth and improvement across the entire life span in which communities and social structures and related policies, as well as individuals, have a role to play.

Ultimately, all ideas of successful aging include being free of physical and cognitive disease and disability. However, when it comes to social engagement, the updated thinking on the topic considers an individual's history and subjective inner satisfaction versus an objective or standardized fixed definition of what success looks like. The takeaway: When it comes to your personal happiness, don't compare yourself to others. For example, actually feeling a positive social connection with others is more important than the simple measure of whether you attend a weekly hobby class.

CHAPTER 2

THE BAD NEWS FIRST

The relationship between telomere length and disease may be a two-way street. To some extent, shorter telomeres result in cellular dysfunction that can lead to disease. In a recent meta-analysis of dozens of studies on heart disease and diabetes, shorter telomeres increased the risk for both. On the other hand, the known oxidative stress and inflammation caused by heart disease, obesity, insulin resistance, smoking, pollution, not exercising enough, psychological stress, or an unhealthful diet are linked to prematurely shorter telomeres.

OBESITY, DIABETES, CANCER, AND OTHER DISEASE STATES

OBESITY

Obesity may contribute to accelerated telomere shortening because of increased oxidative stress and chronic inflammation. A meta-analysis of 87 observational studies that captured data from more than 146,000 adults found that a higher body mass index (BMI) was associated with shorter telomeres over-all, especially in adults ages 18 to 60. For every 5 points higher that a BMI score climbed beyond normal weight (BMI of 25), a person's telomeres were shortened to the equivalent of an additional year of aging. The findings held true for both men and women. The lesson here may be to address obesity before it leads to the onset of disease, providing us with an earlier target for prevention.

Interestingly, there was no relationship between obesity, telomere length, and mortality in the elderly (ages 75 and older). This may be because BMI better reflects body fat in younger people. In older people, muscle loss is an issue, and an individual is more likely to have low muscle and high fat at a lower BMI—that is, more fat per mass. This is a good reminder not to judge a book by its cover, or someone's health status by their weight alone. Thin on the outside, fat on the inside (TOFI) is a real phenomenon.

Obesity itself may not be the issue but a sign: obesity increases the hormone leptin, which normally inhibits hunger but can be unusually high in obese individuals, leading to leptin resistance; obesity also decreases adiponectin, a hormone that improves insulin sensitivity. Both increases in leptin and decreases in adiponectin are associated with oxidative stress and low-grade inflammation.

Abdominal adiposity, more commonly known as "belly fat," is associated with shorter telomeres. Research reports that gaining weight to the point of obesity speeds up the shortening of telomeres and the process of aging. On the flip side, one study on weight loss and telomeres shows that losing weight can protect telomeres against diminishing and the resulting DNA damage.

TYPE 2 DIABETES

Several studies show that shorter telomeres are associated with insulin resistance and type 2 diabetes. But that doesn't tell us whether insulin resistance and diabetes are shortening telomeres (a common theory) or whether the reverse is true. One study recruited 338 pairs of twins and studied them for more than a decade to look for the answer. Twins are fascinating to study because they inherently remove so many of variables, making the results all the more compelling. In this study, the baseline insulin resistance and telomeres of adult twins in their thirties were measured. Twelve years later, the researchers found that the shorter the telomeres were at baseline, the greater the insulin resistance more than a decade later. These results were in addition to any effect weight had on increasing insulin resistance.

While this study suggests that people who start adulthood with shorter telomeres are more likely to develop insulin resistance, that doesn't make it destiny. There are many age-related and environmental factors that can lead to insulin resistance. The best defense is an offense made up of healthy habits.

CANCER

The relationship between telomeres and cancer is complicated. There seems to be a strong link between shorter telomeres and a risk for bladder and stomach cancers, but not breast or other cancers. In contrast, longer telomeres are associated with an increased risk for melanoma, sarcoma, lymphoma, and lung cancer—suggesting they keep some cells around for too long and they don't die off as they should, leading to cancers. There is risk at both extremes.

CHRONIC FATIGUE SYNDROME

The cause of chronic fatigue syndrome (CFS), also called myalgic encephalomyelitis (ME), is unknown. Many symptoms resemble accelerated aging. A study used telomeres as a marker for aging to see if this was true. Indeed, results showed a link between the condition and premature telomere shortening in females younger than 45.

CHRONIC KIDNEY DISEASE

Interestingly, the longer someone has chronic kidney disease is not directly related to shorter and shorter telomeres. There is a U-shaped, or nonlinear, relationship between telomere length and the duration of chronic kidney disease. That is, while one might expect telomeres to get shorter the longer someone lives with a disease, that is not always the case. Researchers think that chronic oxidative stress and inflammation, in some cases, may activate mechanisms that cause telomeres to lengthen. This happens in particular conditions and we're still learning why certain disease states act this way.

GENETIC DISORDERS THAT AFFECT TELOMERES

Short telomere syndromes are conditions related to telomeres that unravel too quickly. They may be linked to a mutation in any of 13 genes known to produce a cluster of proteins that maintain telomere development, length, and stability. Short telomeres, at clinically relevant levels, can be used to diagnose short telomere syndrome; 90% of cases are in adults.

Overly short telomeres inhibit stem cell growth, making it harder to grow, develop, and heal normally. Cells that divide often, such as bone marrow, and skin and inner linings (epithelia) are most at risk. Mutations in telomerase and telomere genes are the most common causes of genetically inherited bone marrow failure.

SLEEP

There is an established relationship between getting older and poor sleep. There is a research-backed association between not getting enough sleep and inflammation, oxidative stress, decreased ability to lower blood pressure during sleep, and disruptions in how the brain regulates hormones.

Insomnia (sleeping less than 6 hours) and sleeping longer than 8 hours were each associated with short telomeres, according to a 2018 study of 925 adults observed overnight in a sleep lab. Short telomeres were defined as telomeres that were in the bottom 10% of the distribution of telomere lengths in the study population.

The results are not as clear-cut when it comes to one of the most common sleep disorders, obstructive sleep apnea (OSA). More than 20 million adults in the United States suffer from OSA, a breathing disorder that causes breathing to stop and start during sleep when throat muscles relax and block the airway. This is what leads to snoring.

The case of OSA and telomeres is a perfect example that challenges the idea that longer is always better, or that poor health always leads to shorter telomeres. The relationship is not always linear.

On the one hand, several well-controlled studies have shown that moderate to severe OSA is related to telomere shortening. On the other hand, a recent study found this to be true only in people with mild OSA and actually found telomere lengthening in people with moderate to severe OSA. The researchers noted that this trend has also been seen in children and that the relationship needs further study. They speculated about their results, citing research showing that telomerase increases in endothelial cells in low-oxygen, or hypoxemic, conditions. It's also possible for telomerase to selectively lengthen short telomeres in acidic (low pH) environments. Both acidic and hypoxic environments are part of OSA. Perhaps relatedly, telomeres lengthen in several cancers when telomerase activity is triggered, and research suggests that OSA may increase the risk of cancer. This study may present a clue to how that works. That said, this was a cross-sectional study so it only captured a moment in time and did not measure blood levels of telomerase. Additional research is needed to prove these mechanisms.

Poor sleep can also affect telomeres in the young, putting them at increased risk for health issues, according to the Fragile Families and Child Wellbeing Study, which included 1,567 children as young as age 9. A review of 19 papers (reduced from an original skimming of nearly 400 papers) found that mothers with sleep apnea had children whose telomeres were already short at age 2.

A study of 176 adults found that multiple aspects of good sleep were each associated with longer telomeres. In contrast, those who took longer to fall asleep and slept for a shorter time had shorter telomeres.

In a 2018 study, insomnia that led to less than 6 hours of sleep had the strongest association with short telomeres. This type of insomnia was also linked to an increased risk for diabetes, cognitive impairment, depression, high blood pressure, and cardiovascular diseases. Insomnia activates stress and immune systems, and now we are learning that it also leads to short telomeres. However, self-reported poor sleepers without insomnia disorders did not have the same short telomeres, but self-reported oversleepers did.

A meta-analysis study that reviewed eight studies involving a total of 2,639 people found that OSA was significantly related to shortened telomeres. Knowing that people with OSA have shorter telomeres means we know they could benefit from preventive care programs for telomere health.

STRESS

Stress comes in many varieties. While we can't control many of the things in life that may bring us stress, we can manage how we react to it (see Stress Management, page 98, for helpful ideas for how to do just that). This chapter discusses the kinds of stress that have been connected to telomere health in the scientific literature.

CAREGIVING

Early work studying stress and telomeres found that the stress of caring for a chronically disabled family member led to psychosocial stress, which, in turn, led to premature aging evidenced by shorter telomeres. However, a 2019 study of 1,233 adults in Cebu, Philippines, found no link between telomere length and the duration of caregiving, relationship to the chronically ill person, or caregiver age and sex. The U.S.-based Nurses' Health Study, which studied a similar size group (1,250 women) had similar findings in 2018. The study authors hypothesized that it is possible that specific kinds of severe caregiving stress could shorten telomere length, but that not all caregiving does so.

PRENATAL STRESS

A mother's stress during pregnancy may impact telomere length starting in the womb. The theory is that an unborn child's initial telomere length setting is changeable during development and can be impacted by challenges to the pregnant woman's immune and endocrine systems, as well as her ability to handle oxidative stress. Stress can come from a variety of sources, including metabolic, social, environmental, and clinical (e.g., fetal growth restriction, diabetes, preeclampsia).

A study of zebra finches found that having shorter telomeres early in life was a strong predictor of a shorter life span. Another animal study, this time of chickens, found that giving hens the stress hormone cortisol meant their offspring had more short telomeres. In humans, emerging science found that severe psychosocial stress during pregnancy added 3.5 years of cellular aging to babies. A smaller study found that pregnancy-related stress (e.g., worrying about the pregnancy itself) influenced the newborn's telomere length by up to 25%.

CHILDHOOD STRESS

Childhood adversity affects children's telomeres in the moment of adversity, but with longer-term effects too. In a systematic study of childhood adversity and telomeres in children ages 3 to 15, researchers found signs of premature cellular aging early in life. Childhood stress was defined as exposure to violence, poverty, a mother's depression, family disruption (e.g., divorce), and institutionalization.

In another study, of children 5 to 10 years old, researchers found that exposure to two or more types of violence manifested in stress-related premature shortening of telomeres over the five-year study period. The types of violence ranged from maternal domestic violence, to frequent bullying, to physical abuse by an adult (this measure included hitting by a parent or their romantic partner, beating by a young adult step-sibling, and sexual abuse). It is upsetting that this kind of childhood stress even exists, and adds insult to injury that it has long-term effects on a child's outlook for a healthy life.

POST-TRAUMATIC STRESS DISORDER (PTSD)

A 2019 study demonstrated that PTSD patients have shorter overall telomeres compared with healthy people. This study was done in an Armenian population, but these findings are in line with previous research in other populations.

CHRONIC SOCIAL STRESS

This type of stress is defined as coming from poverty, exposure to violence, or family caregiving. Chronic stress from social sources, that is, from our families and communities, is associated with telomere shortening whether the exposure to these kinds of stressors happens during childhood or adulthood, according to a systematic review published in *Aging Research Reviews*. There are only a few dozen studies in this area, most of them snapshots of a moment in time (cross-sectional study design) and only a few following people for longer periods (longitudinal studies). The studies examined different stressors or measured telomeres differently. Therefore, it is difficult to definitively link chronic social stress to shorter telomeres, but the evidence is suggestive that chronic stressors cause people to biologically age faster. More research is needed, but in the meantime there are many reasons to alleviate chronic social stress.

POOR RELATIONSHIPS

A 2018 study found that poor interpersonal relationships were associated with higher stress levels and shorter telomeres. The study included more than 200 people who self-reported their levels of attachment to others and their stress levels. Poor outcomes were linked to being overly attached and to avoiding attachment; both were unhealthful. This is a new way to see how close relationships can impact health and aging.

LONG-TERM VS. SHORT-TERM

Long-term stress seems to have a damaging effect on telomere health, perhaps through spikes of cortisol, the body's main stress hormone. A 2019 meta-analysis reviewed 14 studies that looked at cortisol and telomere length. Specific instances of stress that spiked cortisol were associated with shorter telomeres, especially in children and female adults.

The silver lining is that one stressful situation on its own doesn't seem to do lasting damage to telomeres, as long as it doesn't become the source of chronic stress. This means that developing ways to respond well to stress may help with telomere health, as well as more immediate everyday feelings of well-being.

TOBACCO

It is well known, and confirmed by the Centers for Diseases Control and Prevention (CDC), that cigarette smoking harms every organ of the body, and quitting can add years to a person's life. Smoking tobacco produces oxidative stress and inflammation that, as expected, is reflected in telomere shortening. In a study of women, for every pack-year (equivalent to smoking a 20-cigarette pack per day for a year), lost an additional 18% of their telomeres compared to the overall sample, equivalent to 7.4 years of life over a 40-year period. In a cross-sectional snapshot study of a day in the life of 477 generally healthy volunteers ages 20 to 50 years, all smokers had shorter telomeres compared with people who had never smoked.

The relationship between secondhand smoke and telomeres has not been well studied, but other very well-documented health consequences provide more than enough reasons to avoid secondhand smoke, such as more severe asthma, ear infections, respiratory distress, and infections in children, and a greater risk for heart disease, lung cancer, and stroke in adults.

IRON

Iron is an important part of hemoglobin, the protein that transfers oxygen from the lungs to the rest of the body's tissues. It's also part of myoglobin, the protein that provides oxygen to muscles. However, people with iron levels that are too high tend to have shorter telomeres than people with normal iron levels. This is according to new findings from the National Health and Nutrition Examination Survey (NHANES), which looked at a link between iron and telomere length in more than 7,000 adults.

Extra iron stores have the potential to create an environment of oxidative stress in the body, especially in adults age 65 years and older. Older adults create fewer antioxidants to combat the oxidative stress that extra iron could promote, making food sources of antioxidants even more important.

Previous research has found that iron supplements increase free radical formation. Iron intake from food or low-iron multivitamins have not been linked to shorter telomeres. As the Renaissance physician Paracelsus said, "Only the dose makes the poison." This holds true for iron. Amounts found naturally in foods raise very little risk of iron overload, but excessive levels made possible by supplements may raise the risk for greater oxidative stress and telomere shortening.

In addition, side effects can be felt after just one large dose. Twenty mg/kg of iron supplements (e.g., 1,361 mg for a 150-pound person) can lead to constipation, nausea, vomiting, abdominal pain, faintness, and stomach upset. The recommended upper limit is 40 to 45 mg per day.

Supplemental Iron Upper Limit

AGE	AMOUNT
Birth to 13 years	40 mg
14+ years	45 mg
Pregnant or lactating: 45 mg	

Source: Institute of Medicine, Food and Nutrition Board, Dietary Reference Intakes

A healthy intake of the heme form of iron, from animal foods such as seafood and poultry, is just 18 mg per day, as noted in the Daily Value (DV) listed on nutrition labels. Individual needs vary by life stage, as shown in the table below.

Recommended Heme Iron per Day

AGE	MALE	FEMALE
Birth to 6 months	0.27 mg	0.27 mg
7–12 months	11 mg	11 mg
1–3 years	7 mg	7 mg
4–8 years	10 mg	10 mg
9–13 years	8 mg	8 mg
14–18 years	11 mg	15 mg 27 mg (pregnant) 10 mg (lactating)
19–50 years	8 mg	18 mg 27 mg (pregnant) 9 mg (lactating)
51+ years	8 mg	8 mg

Source: Institute of Medicine, Food and Nutrition Board, Dietary Reference Intakes

An adjusted recommended intake for vegetarians is 1.8 times higher due to a lower rate of bioavailability of the nonheme form of iron, which comes from plant foods and supplements, including the form used in fortified foods. Healthy plant-based sources of iron include nuts, beans, and vegetables. Vitamin C, seafood, and poultry all help the body absorb nonheme iron. For example, to get more of the nonheme iron from baby spinach, simply toss some orange segments or slices of bell pepper, or use a lemon vinaigrette (all sources of vitamin C) on a baby spinach salad.

While it's true that some compounds, such as certain phytates and polyphenols in beans and other foods, can inhibit nonheme iron absorption, and calcium may reduce the bioavailability of both heme and nonheme iron, the effects are minimal in the context of a typical varied diet and have little impact on iron status. As long as you're eating a balanced diet, you don't need to be overly concerned.

Recommended Nonheme Iron per Day for Vegetarians

AGE	MALE	FEMALE
Birth to 6 months	0.49 mg	0.49 mg
7–12 months	20 mg	20 mg
1–3 years	13 mg	13 mg
4–8 years	18 mg	18 mg
9–13 years	14 mg	14 mg
14–18 years	20 mg	27 mg 49 mg (pregnant) 18 mg (lactating)
19–50 years	14 mg	32 mg 49 mg (pregnant) 16 mg (lactating)
51+ years	14 mg	14 mg

Source: Institute of Medicine, Food and Nutrition Board, Dietary Reference Intakes

Below are examples of healthy foods that can be incorporated into meals and snacks to meet your iron needs.

Iron Food Sources

FOOD	AMOUNT	% DV
Oysters, 3 ounces cooked	18 mg	44%
White beans, canned, 1 cup	8 mg	44%
Dark chocolate, 45%–69% cacao, 3 ounces	7 mg	39%
Lentils, ½ cup cooked	3 mg	17%
Spinach, ½ cup cooked	3 mg	17%
Firm tofu, ½ cup	3 mg	17%
Kidney beans, canned, ½ cup	2 mg	11%
Bone-in sardines, canned, 3 ounces	2 mg	11%
Chickpeas, ½ cup cooked	2 mg	11%
Tomatoes, stewed, canned, ½ cup	2 mg	11%
Baked potato with skin, medium	2 mg	11%
Green peas, ½ cup cooked	1 mg	6%
Whole wheat bread, 1 slice	1 mg	6%
Raisins, ¼ cup	1 mg	6%
Whole wheat spaghetti, 1 cup cooked	1 mg	6%
Pistachios, 1 ounce (49 nuts)	1 mg	6%
Broccoli, ½ cup cooked	1 mg	6%
Egg, 1 large, hard-boiled	1 mg	6%

Source: USDA National Nutrient Database for Standard Reference Legacy Release

*The Daily Value (DV) used for these calculations is 18 mg.

DIET PATTERNS
FOR POOR HEALTH

Studies on total diet and telomeres are based largely on observational data. The research shows a relationship between poor telomere health and the same dietary patterns that lead to poor health outcomes. Namely, excessive total and saturated fats, refined grains, meat and meat products, and sugar-sweetened beverages were linked to shorter telomeres.

Telomere length may be sensitive to long-term intake of sugar-sweetened beverages. In a study of 5,309 generally healthy U.S. adults ages 20 to 65, sugar-sweetened beverage drinkers had shorter telomeres. So far, no association has been found between diet soda and telomeres, although a recent study linked diet drinks sweetened with artificial sweeteners to a 23% increased risk of stroke via blocked small arteries in post-menopausal women who had two artificially sweetened diet drinks a day.

Data on dairy and alcohol are mixed, and a moderation approach is advisable given some of the health benefits associated with intake of these foods. Research findings on a link between alcohol and telomeres are mixed. A cross-sectional study of nearly 500 healthy adults ages 20 to 50 years found no relationship between drinking alcohol and telomere length.

On the one hand, the Mediterranean diet, one of the best-studied healthy diets, allows for a glass of polyphenol-rich wine with meals. This is in line with the Dietary Guidelines for Americans to drink in moderation if at all—up to one drink per day for women and two for men.

On the other hand, there are people who should not drink at all. They include people who are pregnant, underage, recovering alcoholics, or at risk for certain kinds of cancer (e.g., breast cancer, esophageal cancer, head and neck cancer). In a study of 200 drunk drivers diagnosed as alcohol abusers, the telomere length of these subjects were nearly half the length of the control, or comparison, group made up of 257 social drinkers. Alcohol abusers drank more than four drinks a day. This study didn't include nondrinkers, but it's interesting to see that social drinkers fared better than alcohol abusers, which is one more indication that moderation is key.

Alcohol is a tricky part of the diet. Overdoing it is definitely harmful, and you certainly don't need to drink wine to get polyphenols, but if you enjoy wine or any other alcohol from time to time, the best advice is to do so in reasonable amounts as recommended by health experts. Cheers!

CHAPTER 3

NOW THE GOOD NEWS

It is estimated that up to 50% of telomere length is inherited. But genes are not destiny. We have quite a bit of power and influence over our own well-being. In fact, research of twins suggests that 80% of how long and how well we live depends on variables like nutrition and lifestyle. While this means there's more work for each one of us to do to improve our own well-being, this is good news. It means we have a significant say in how successfully we age.

The solution is an anti-inflammatory, antioxidant-rich, and fiber-rich plant-based diet, along with smart limitations on the things that create or worsen the effects of inflammation and oxidative stress. The kind of eating pattern that helps maintain and even lengthen telomeres is one that celebrates vegetables, fruit, nuts, olive oil, and fish, and can even include a glass of red wine now and then (excessive alcohol has the opposite effect). Getting 20 minutes of exercise three times a week helps support a happy healthy body as well.

DIET PATTERNS
FOR TELOMERE HEALTH

MEDITERRANEAN DIET

Consistently ranked by experts as one of the healthiest diet patterns, the Mediterranean diet is backed by decades of positive research findings and centuries of tradition. The eating pattern is based on seasonal fruits and vegetables, nuts and seeds, whole grains, olive oil, fish, and low-fat meat, with smaller amounts of dairy and alcohol (mostly wine). In the Nurses' Health Study, a subset of 4,700 disease-free women who most closely followed the Mediterranean diet were able to stave off telomere shortening to the equivalent of 4.5 fewer years of aging. The protective effect of the Mediterranean diet that kept these women 4.5 years biologically younger is the reverse of the negative impact of smoking (4.6 years of aging) and inactivity (4.4 years of aging).

The key to the Mediterranean eating pattern may be its anti-oxidant and anti-inflammatory potential. A small study of 20 men and women 65 years and older tested the theory. The study had the group eat according to one of the following plans for a month: the Mediterranean diet, a low-fat/high-carb diet, or a diet higher in saturated fat. The people following the Mediterranean diet saw improvements in oxidative stress markers and telomere shortening compared with their status when they started on the diet, and compared with people on the other two diets.

One of the ways the eating pattern could be working is by improving telomerase activity. In addition, components of the Mediterranean diet have been shown to lower oxidative stress markers and inflammation. Here's the evidence.

A large-scale study of the Mediterranean diet, dubbed PREDIMED (Primary Prevention of Cardiovascular Disease with a

Mediterranean Diet), found that people who started the five-year study with longer telomeres lost more weight and had a lower body mass index (BMI) and less belly fat (waist circumference) after following a Mediterranean diet that included extra-virgin olive oil and nuts.

This is great news for people who are interested in eating the Mediterranean way and have either already been following a healthy lifestyle to maintain their telomeres, are lucky enough to have inherited longer telomeres, or some combination of the two. The good news for the rest of us is that the effect went both ways. Over those same five years of the study, the people who lost weight also increased their telomere length. The average age of the more than 500 adults in this study was 67 years, showing that it's never too late to make healthy changes.

WHAT'S SO SPECIAL ABOUT THE MEDITERRANEAN DIET?

A 2019 review study took a deeper dive into the functional components of the Mediterranean diet to better understand how it keeps telomeres healthy.

- Olive oil: Polyphenols, healthy monounsaturated fats, and antioxidant vitamin E

- Beans and legumes: Polyphenols

- Whole grains and potatoes: Vitamins, minerals, polyphenols, and fiber

- Vegetables: Polyphenols, organosulfurs, phytosterols, and carotenoids

- Fruit: Polyphenols, antioxidants, and minerals

- Nuts: Healthy fats, fiber, polyphenols, and minerals

- Wine: Resveratrol and other polyphenols

- Dairy: Probiotics

- Seafood: Omega-3 fatty acids

This review study made it clear that the strength of the Mediterranean diet may be the synergy of a great variety of bioactive nutrients from diverse food groups. The whole of the diet pattern may be protecting telomeres more than any one component alone. Nutrients often work together in ways we don't yet fully understand. Indeed, the diet pattern has already been shown to prevent, manage, and treat heart disease, diabetes, and cognitive decline, and improve feelings of well-being.

VEGETARIAN DIETS

A plant-based diet such as a vegetarian diet can often lead to health benefits. However, the research on vegetarian diets—including variations with eggs and dairy—is unclear, and no significant changes to telomere length have been seen to date. Some research shows vegetarian diets are higher in antioxidants and lower in fat, but also lower in vitamins B and D as well as iron and calcium. Different studies show conflicting results for overall health, antioxidant status, and DNA damage.

Does this mean vegetarian diets aren't healthy? Not at all. What it likely means is that the term "vegetarian" is too broad and that there is more to health outcomes than simply the avoidance of meat. That is, the quality of all the other nonmeat foods in the diet matters just as much. For example, potato chips can be just as vegetarian as a kale and chickpea salad, but they obviously contain different nutrients.

Because a vegetarian diet removes food groups, it takes more planning to ensure that all nutrient needs are being met—but it is definitely doable.

OUR FIRST DIET PATTERN

Breast milk is the preferred first food for infants. Think of it as our first healthy eating pattern, simple though it may be as it's just one food. The American Academy of Pediatrics recommends exclusively breastfeeding for the first six months, with only the addition of vitamin D unless another course is medically recommended. Even shorter periods seem to be helpful when it comes to telomeres, according to a study that found that infants exclusively breastfed for the first four to six weeks of life had longer telomeres at ages 4 and 5.

CALORIE RESTRICTION

The research on calorie restriction and telomere health in humans is in its infancy, but the findings in favor of restricting calories suggests possible health benefits even if the impact on telomeres is not yet clear.

There are very few studies on calorie restriction and telomere length or telomerase activity in humans, although benefits are clearly demonstrated in rodent studies. Three studies involving diverse human populations did not find any significant relationship between calories and telomeres. One study found a different result, but it was in a younger population of males only, ages 30 to 43.

The first randomized human trial studying a 25% calorie restriction showed physiological benefits. The six-month trial resulted in a 10% weight loss including visceral fat, subcutaneous fat, and muscle. Improvements were also demonstrated through reduced fasting insulin concentrations, lower triglycerides, an increase in better-for-you high-density lipoprotein cholesterol (HDL cholesterol), and lower total cholesterol and blood pressure, all leading to a 28% lower risk for heart disease. However, by the end of the trial, participants reported feelings of increased hunger and appetite, suggesting it may not be a sustainable strategy.

A smaller calorie reduction may be more feasible. Consider that Okinawans, many of whom live past 100 years, eat a well-balanced diet that has about 15% to 20% fewer calories than the diets of their fellow citizens in the rest of Japan. Okinawans eat about 40% less than the average American adult. There is a term from Confucian teaching, *hara hachi bun me*, that roughly translates to "eat until you are 80 percent full," which helps explain their approach to eating.

As always, the quality of calories matters. Unintended consequences of focusing on restriction include an unhealthy relationship with food and, in this dietitian's opinion, is not the best approach. Improving the quality of the diet by focusing on healthy foods to eat can often have a side effect of calorie reduction without overengineering the restriction aspect.

WHAT IS INTERMITTENT FASTING?

Intermittent fasting (IF) is a kind of calorie restriction, with many variations in how it's done.

- The 16/8 method: Don't eat for 14 to 16 hours, which leaves 8 to 10 hours open for nourishment. The 16/8 method most closely mimics a normal eating pattern.

- 5:2 plan: Eat as you normally would for five days in a row, then eat only 500 to 600 calories a day in the next two days.

- Eat-stop diet: Fast for 24 hours a couple of times a week. This is similar to alternate-day fasting, which is exactly what it sounds like.

- Warrior diet: Starve during the day and eat one huge meal in the evening. This is a feast and famine kind of regimen.

IF has gained popular attention, but the research in people is less clear about its benefits. The evidence for IF-driven weight loss varies quite a bit, and most studies show no significant weight loss or even improvement in metabolic markers. We don't yet know if it's safe for all ages or all health statuses, or if there are negative health consequences, especially for those with preexisting conditions. We also don't know how it helps or hurts exercise, and what the optimal foods are, because right now IF is all about timing and calories.

HEALTHY EATING PATTERNS

There is no doubt that the Mediterranean diet is one of the best-studied healthy eating patterns. It's reasonable to wonder how other evidence-backed healthy patterns support telomere health. A 2018 study reviewed data from 4,758 U.S. adults ages 20 to 65 to find out. They were a generally healthy, nationally representative group of people. The study scored a day's worth of eating according to how well it matched recommendations from four evidence-based healthy eating patterns: Healthy Eating Index 2010, Alternate Healthy Eating Index 2010, Mediterranean diet, and Dietary Approaches to Stop Hypertension (DASH). Scores were split into five tiers, and the top tier in any of the eating patterns had significantly longer telomeres than the bottom tier, at least in women; this was equivalent to three to four years of aging. The researchers weren't sure why the effect was not seen in men, other than a trend toward longer telomeres in men on the DASH diet.

While the various diets have some unique differences, what they have in common are high intakes of fruit, vegetables, whole grains, dairy foods, and plant-based proteins, and lower intakes of red meat, processed meat, sodium, and added sugars.

U.S. Healthy Eating Patterns

EATING PATTERN	SCORE	ATTRIBUTES THAT ADD TO THE SCORE	ATTRIBUTES THAT DIMINISH THE SCORE
Healthy Eating Index (HEI) 2010 Based on: *2010 Dietary Guidelines for Americans*	Best: 100 Average: 46.3	Total fruit intake Choosing whole fruit Total vegetable intake Eating leafy greens Beans Whole grains Dairy Total protein food intake Seafood and plant proteins Fatty acids	Refined grains Sodium Empty calories
Alternate Healthy Eating Index (AHEI) 2010 Based on: *Harvard School of Public Health's Healthy Eating Plate*	Best: 110 Average: 37	Vegetables Fruits Whole grains Nuts and legumes Long-chain fats Polyunsaturated fats Moderate alcohol intake	Sugar-sweetened beverages and fruit juices Red/processed meats Trans fat, and sodium
Mediterranean diet Based on: *Mediterranean diet adapted for the U.S.*	Best: 55 Average: 21	Whole grains Fruits, vegetables Potatoes Legumes Fish Monounsaturated fats Moderate consumption of alcohol	Red meat Poultry Full-fat dairy

U.S. Healthy Eating Patterns

EATING PATTERN	SCORE	ATTRIBUTES THAT ADD TO THE SCORE	ATTRIBUTES THAT DIMINISH THE SCORE
Dietary Approaches to Stop Hypertension (DASH) **Based on:** *Developed by the National Heart, Lung, and Blood Institute to prevent and control hypertension*	Best: 40 Average: 23.9	Fruit Vegetables Nuts and legumes Whole grains Low-fat dairy	Sodium Red meat Processed meat Sugar-sweetened beverages

FOODS FOR TELOMERE HEALTH

WHOLE GRAINS

Fiber, particularly the fiber in whole grains, was significantly associated with longer telomeres in a cross-sectional study of nearly 2,300 women participating in the Nurses' Health Study. The participants were in their fifties and sixties when their telomere length was measured.

Whole grains are grains whose three original components— bran, endosperm, and germ—remain intact and at the same levels as when the grains were growing in the fields. The bran is the outer skin. Think of it like the skin on sweet potatoes, apples, or pears: edible and full of antioxidants, B vitamins, and fiber. The fleshy endosperm is where the nutrients for the developing seed are stored, and it's usually made up of starch and other nutrients. The germ is the embryo, which, under the right conditions, has the potential to sprout into a new plant.

NUTS

A study of more than 5,500 U.S. adults from the National Health and Nutrition Examination Survey (NHANES) found that eating nuts and seeds slowed down biological aging on a cellular level. The relationship was linear: the more nuts and seeds eaten, the greater the benefit to telomere length. For each 1% of total calories that came from nuts and seeds, telomeres were five base pairs longer. This study found that among adults of the same chronological age, people who got 5% of their calories from nuts and seeds were biologically 1.5 years younger than their peers.

Let's do some quick math. If you average 2,000 calories per day, then 5% of your calories equals 100 calories, which works out to about 14 almonds (7 calories per nut), 29 pistachios (3.5 calories per kernel), 67 pumpkin seeds (1.5 calories per seed), or a little more than 4 teaspoons of chia seeds (23 calories per teaspoon).

Most of the research on nuts and seeds is on nuts, so I'll discuss the nut research and we'll assume that seeds have a similar nutrient profile, including healthy fats and antioxidant benefits. Also, most tree nut research in the United States also includes peanuts because of their similar nutrient profile and use in the American diet, even though they are technically a legume.

From research released by Harvard University in 2013, we learned that eating tree nuts every day is associated with a healthier life span and 20% reduced risk of dying from all causes but especially heart disease (29% risk reduction) and cancer (11% risk reduction). The more often people ate nuts, the greater the benefit. Again, the relationship between the dose of nuts and health span benefit was linear. For example, snacking on nuts once a week reduced risk by 11% overall, and at five times a week the risk was reduced by 15%. Eating nuts seven times a week or more had the greatest benefit (20% risk reduction).

Nuts and seeds are valuable sources of plant-based dietary fiber, protein, healthy fats, and essential micronutrients, vitamins, and minerals. In addition to their emerging role in telomere health, they help keep your heart, immune system, digestive tract, blood sugar, satiety, and bones healthy.

Tree nuts include almonds, Brazil nuts, cashews, hazelnuts, macadamia nuts, pecans, pistachios, pine nuts, and walnuts. Most of the research on the health benefits of individual nuts has been conducted on almonds, pistachios, and walnuts. Nuts make excellent snacks on their own, in trail mixes, or in recipes. Examples of seeds include chia seeds, flax seeds (also called linseeds), pepitas (pumpkin seeds), perilla seeds, poppy seeds, sesame seeds, and sunflower seeds. Some seeds, such as sunflower seeds, lend themselves to snacking, but most are used in recipes.

NUTTY SPOTLIGHT: WALNUTS

A 2019 study found that polyphenols in walnuts reduced telomerase activity in colon cancer cells, in a dose-dependent manner. Telomere length in cancer cells decreased along with dampened telomerase activity. This study was the next logical step after an earlier study found that walnut polyphenols could threaten colon cancer stem cells. Recall that telomerase is especially active in cancer cells and stem cells, but not in most normal cells. These were both cell studies that hinted at the anticancer benefits of eating walnuts, but additional research is needed to confirm results in humans. That said, there are plenty of well-established heart health and general healthy eating benefits to including walnuts in snacks and meals.

LEGUMES

Legumes such as beans, chickpeas, lentils, peas, broad beans, peanuts, and soybeans contain phytochemicals that might dampen the activity of telomerase in select cancer cells. Legumes contain flavonoids such as apigenin, quercetin, daidzein, and kaempferol. Flavonoids are a large class of nutrients known for their antioxidant and anti-inflammatory properties, and for giving plant foods their color. Chickpeas, for example, contain the isoflavone genisten, which may inhibit telomerase at high intakes.

The connection between legumes and telomeres has not been well studied to date. However, a 2015 study of nearly 2,000 middle-aged Korean adults found that those who ate more legumes had healthier telomere lengths. These findings were similar to a small 2015 study in a young male Spanish population. The significance is that benefits were seen in different age groups and ethnicities, suggesting there is a universal benefit. However, several observational studies have not yet been able to show any significant association between legumes and telomere length.

SEAFOOD

Fish and seaweed provide the heart- and brain-healthy omega-3 fats EPA and DHA (see Omega-3s section, page 80) that are hard to get from food. So it is no wonder that both of these foods were associated with longer and healthier telomeres in a 10-year study of 1,958 older Korean adults. The results were based on eating patterns established a decade prior to telomeres being measured. In so many cases of nutrition impacting longevity and health span, we see time and again that everyday habits over many years can help or harm our health.

In a Harvard study that didn't look at telomeres but did look at the risk of premature death, older adults with the highest levels of omega-3s from fish lived, on average, 2.2 years longer. Plus, based on 26 different studies that included a total of 150,278 people, eating more fish reduced the risk of depression in both males and females. Depression is linked with shorter telomeres.

Eating seafood two to three times a week helps people live more years in good health, reducing the risk of premature death by 17%. According to the most recently available report from the National Oceanic and Atmospheric Administration (NOAA), released in late 2018, fish consumption went up 3.6% in 2017, with Americans eating on average 16 pounds in 2017 versus 14.9 pounds in 2016. That's 256 ounces per year, or 64 servings, which averages out to 1.2 servings a week. That's good, but there's room to grow.

The most commonly consumed fish in the United States are:

1. Shrimp

2. Salmon

3. Canned tuna

4. Tilapia

5. Alaska pollock

6. Pangasius (basa or swai)

7. Cod

8. Crab

9. Catfish

10. Clams

These are a good place to start, but when you're ready to add some diversity to the seafood on your plate, check out the top fish by omega-3s (see the table on page 81).

GREEN TEA

Green tea contains a polyphenol called epigallocatechin gallate (EGCG), which has anti-inflammatory and antioxidant properties. In a small study, green tea supplementation for eight weeks lengthened telomeres in obese women, even without weight loss. That said, there is generally an inverse relationship between telomere length and BMI, which measures body fat as a ratio of weight to height. The study's control group consisted of women of normal weight; their telomeres were significantly longer at baseline, even before the study started. Because there was no weight loss, the study's findings suggest it was the effect of the green tea alone, independent of any relationship between lower weight and longer telomeres. The study participants took a supplement with approximately 900 mg EGCG per day for eight weeks.

That dosage (900 mg EGCG) equates to 4 to 18 cups of green tea per day, according to a comparison of eight different green teas. The amount of EGCG ranged from 50 mg (Stash Premium brand) to 238 mg (Celestial Seasoning) per cup. It's worth noting that the comparison did not include matcha green tea, which another study suggests has at least three times the EGCG as the highest published value in regular green tea, putting it at around 700 mg EGCG per cup.

In an observational study of regular tea drinkers in China, elderly Chinese men 65 years and older who drank 3 cups a day had longer telomeres than those who only had 1 cup per week. Their longer telomeres equated to approximately five additional years of life.

The majority of health research on tea is done on true tea made from *Camellia sinensis* leaves, which includes white tea, yellow tea (rare), green tea (including matcha tea), oolong tea, dark tea (including pu-erh tea), and black tea. They all come from the same plant but are oxidized to different levels. Black tea is fully oxidized, green and white teas are not oxidized after harvest, and oolong tea is partially oxidized and lies somewhere in between. Dark tea is more of a specialty tea and is fermented. The protective EGCG compound is found in all types of true tea.

This doesn't mean there's anything wrong with herbal teas, which are made from infusions of herbs, spices, and other plants. Examples of herbal teas are chamomile, peppermint, and toasted barley. As you can imagine, there's a greater variety of herbal teas, sometimes called tisanes, than true tea. There are small studies on specific tisanes here and there, and they are certainly a good hydration choice that's calorie-, sugar-, and sodium-free. All the same, it's important to know that the vast majority of health research on tea has been conducted on true tea.

The takeaway: All teas and tisanes are a healthy beverage choice, there is evidence that regular long-term true tea consumption is associated with longer telomeres, and a small study found that green tea in particular can lengthen telomeres in as little as eight weeks.

COFFEE

Coffee lovers will be happy to know that a large study found that as coffee intake increased, so did telomere length, suggesting a speed bump for aging in your morning cup. The observational study included nearly 6,000 men and women ages 20 to 84 across the United States. However, the same study found that caffeine shortened telomere length whether people drank coffee or not. While coffee and caffeine often go hand in hand, the effects of each on telomere length were at odds in this particular study. That's because caffeine is complicated. It has antioxidant properties, although it can also hamper DNA repair, at least in yeast cell studies. It might be that caffeine does indeed shorten telomeres, or that we simply need better data to clearly answer this question. Remember, this was an observational study, so it's hard to draw absolute conclusions about cause and effect.

Nevertheless, the good news is that the connection between coffee intake and longer telomeres persists across other studies.

A study of 4,780 women found that those who drank more regular coffee had longer telomeres despite correspondingly higher caffeine intake. The study did not find any relationship between decaffeinated coffee and telomere length. Researchers speculated that the benefits of coffee outweighed the possible negative effects of caffeine, such as short-term increases in blood pressure, homocysteine (which has been associated with a higher risk of heart disease), and insulin inhibition.

Until we know more, it seems reasonable to stick to the version of coffee that you prefer best, and to stay tuned for more news on caffeine.

100% FRUIT JUICE

One hundred percent fruit juice is associated with longer telomeres. But here's what isn't: sugar-sweetened beverages (including soft drinks, fruit-flavored drinks, sports drinks, and energy drinks) and diet soda. Just because 100% fruit juice is sweet, don't confuse it with sodas or any drinks with added sugar.

Here are tips for finding the best juice:

- The term "100% fruit juice" is regulated. It means the product contains only juice from the whole fruit. Accept nothing else. Read the label. Many juice blends and lemonades may seem to be 100% juice but they're not; such a beverage might be a labeled as a "juice drink," "fruit-flavored drink," or "juice cocktail." Check the ingredients list to see if the product contains any filler juices, added sugar, or added color or preservatives.

- If it says it comes from concentrate, that term on a 100% juice simply means it was reduced down for efficient storage or transportation, and was reconstituted to the original 100% levels. If you see a concentrate in an ingredients list for a food that is not 100% juice, then it is being used as an added sugar. While this is a little complicated, it's important to unpack these nuances so that you aren't unnecessarily avoiding a healthy food like 100% juice.

- The natural color of the juice is a good proxy for polyphenols. For example, Concord grape juice, blueberry juice, tart cherry juice, and pomegranate juice are all deeply hued 100% juices and are all high in antioxidant polyphenols.

- Typically, anything labeled "clarified juice" has been overly processed and possesses fewer complex phytonutrients. Think of the difference between clarified apple juice and unfiltered apple juice, which is cloudy.

ASTRAGALUS

Astragalus is an herb whose thin stringy root is used to make medicine. It has been shown to increase telomerase activity and have antioxidant and anti-inflammatory characteristics. However, well-designed clinical trials are needed to confirm its benefits. While it might sound like an unusual ingredient, it's commonly used in traditional Chinese medicine and contains more than 200 compounds.

One specific component, TA-65, lengthened telomeres in a clinical trial of 117 generally healthy adults ages 53 to 87. A larger study that logged 1,400 peoples' worth of data over five years found that TA-65 was also associated with improved cardiometabolic markers that may indicate a reduced risk of chronic diseases like heart disease, type 2 diabetes, and metabolic syndrome. TA-65 also helps clear out old cells that can impair the immune system.

In experimental models, TA-65 increased telomerase activity in cells with overly short telomeres. It has also lengthened telomeres in a bird model, and increased telomere length via telomerase activation in mouse models. In a study of elderly (2-year-old) female mice, TA-65 administered for four months improved health span, although there were no significant differences in life span. Animal studies suggest that astragalus protects the body's self-made antioxidant superoxide dismutase (SOD) and decreases free radical levels. In a mouse model, it has been shown to increase average telomere length, reduce the percentage of critically short telomeres, and improve DNA repair mechanisms.

Some strains of the herb have been linked to livestock poisonings (e.g., *Astragalus lentiginosus*, *A. mollissimus*), but the kind in dietary supplements is different and is most commonly *A. membranaceus*. Doses up to 60 grams per day have been safely used for four months, according to the *Natural Medicines Comprehensive Database*. It seems to support a healthy immune system and reduce inflammation, but more evidence is needed to prove its clinical benefits. Always talk to your health care team about concerns before using a supplement.

A delicious way to try astragalus in food is in a traditional Korean soup, Samyetang (page 138), which uses several herbs and roots to flavor the broth, often including astragalus root (also known as milk vetch root). The dish is sometimes called ginseng chicken soup, and is thought to have medicinal properties. It's not uncommon for Koreans to have a hot bowl of samyetang when they're feeling under the weather, not unlike chicken soup in the United States.

NUTRIENTS FOR TELOMERE HEALTH

Even though specific nutrients have been studied and found to protect telomeres, a food-first approach ensures you're getting a complex of nutrients that work together in whole foods. The nutrients covered in this section are vitamin A, beta-carotene, lutein, zeaxanthin, vitamin B12, folate, vitamin C, vitamin D, vitamin E, copper, magnesium, zinc, fiber, omega-3 fatty acids, curcumin, and polyphenols.

VITAMIN A AND BETA-CAROTENE

Vitamin A and beta-carotene are associated with healthy telomere length in women who get these nutrients from food but not from supplements. Vitamin A and its precursors (such as beta-carotene) support a healthy immune system that can better fight off infection, a known cause of premature telomere shortening. Indeed, data show that vitamin A deficiency makes a person more prone to infections. In people who were vitamin A deficient, providing vitamin A reduced inflammatory markers and increased anti-inflammatory compounds. However, there does not seem to be a dose-response effect when it comes to telomere health, so more isn't necessarily better.

THE ANTIOXIDANT PARADOX

People who eat plenty of natural sources of beta-carotene, such as fruits and vegetables, have a lower risk of certain cancers, such as lung or prostate cancers. However, the evidence on a benefit for supplementation is not there. To the contrary, smokers taking high doses of beta-carotene supplements are at an increased risk of colon, lung, and prostate cancers.

There are two key things to consider when weighing the benefits of vitamin A in food versus supplements. First, fruits, vegetables, and other foods contain a diversity of nutrients, not just isolated nutrients. Even so, food is more than the sum of its nutrients, and the plant chemicals (aka phytonutrients) in complete food may work synergistically in ways we do not yet fully understand.

Second, it is much more difficult to consume excessive amounts of nutrients in natural foods than it is in supplements.

In a study of older adults, those with more beta-carotene in their circulation—a proxy for how much carotenoid-rich food a person eats—had more active telomerase, the telomere-building enzyme. The study included 68 older adults, consisting of 37 people with Alzheimer's disease in the experimental group and 31 healthy people in the control group. The results were true for both men and women, and were independent of age or whether the person smoked.

Beta-carotene is found in yellow, dark orange, red, and green fruits and vegetables such as carrots, cantaloupe, apricots, sweet potatoes, pumpkin, winter squash (e.g., butternut), mangoes, collard greens, spinach, kale, broccoli, bok choy, turnip greens, mustard greens, dandelion greens, beet greens, and Swiss chard. To make sure you are getting enough vitamin A from foods containing beta-carotene, eat a variety of fruits and vegetables daily. This is much more practical than trying to count all the vitamin A you're getting throughout the day. If more guidance is helpful, aim for at least a total of 2 cups of fruit and 3 cups of vegetables, including both dark green and dark orange ones in the mix.

However, if you are numbers oriented, you should know that beta-carotene is counted in the daily vitamin A recommendation of 900 mcg RAE (retinol activity equivalents). Vitamin A actually refers to a group of nutrients, including beta-carotene and others, that have varying levels of bioactivity measured in micrograms of RAE. The way vitamin A is labeled on foods is going through a transition in 2020–2021, but the label updates will make things simpler to understand. Until then, there are a few things to keep straight.

WHAT IS BETA-CAROTENE?

Beta-carotene is one of more than 600 kinds of carotenoids, antioxidants, and fat-soluble plant pigments responsible for the yellow, orange, and red in fruits and vegetables. It is referred to as provitamin A because the body converts it into vitamin A.

Carotenoid-rich food has antioxidant properties and therefore may be involved in telomere health by reducing oxidative stress. On the flip side, more instances of low beta-carotene intake as measured by levels in the blood have been found in people with Alzheimer's disease compared with people who were cognitively healthy. There's an association of low blood levels of beta-carotene and Alzheimer's disease that remains even after accounting for age, gender, smoking habits, APOE gene type (which can be a genetic marker of risk in certain populations), and telomere length.

Until 2020, vitamin A is allowed to be labeled in international units (IU), which converts to different fractions of micrograms of preformed or provitamin A from foods and supplements. After the change, the various forms of vitamin A will be labeled in micrograms (mcg) RAE. The DV will be 900 mcg RAE. Larger companies have until New Year's Day 2020 to make the change, and smaller companies have one more year, until the start of 2021. For a look at what "1 mcg RAE" on a label equates to, see the table below.

Vitamin A Equivalents

1 MCG RAE	TYPE	SOURCE	EXAMPLES
1 mcg retinol	Preformed vitamin A	Animal	Milk, yogurt, eggs, fish
2 mcg beta-carotene, from supplements	Provitamin A carotenoid	Synthetic	Fortified cereals, supplements

1 MCG RAE	TYPE	SOURCE	EXAMPLES
12 mcg beta-carotene, from food	Provitamin A carotenoid	Plant	Sweet potatoes, carrots, spinach, kale, broccoli, butternut squash
24 mcg alpha-carotene	Provitamin A carotenoid	Plant	Sweet potatoes, carrots, spinach, kale, broccoli, butternut squash
24 mcg beta-cryptoxanthin	Provitamin A carotenoid	Plant	Butternut squash, persimmons, mandarin oranges, sweet red peppers

Women should aim for 700 mcg RAE, and men for 900 mcg RAE. The Daily Value (DV) is changing to 900 mcg RAE, so when you see on a food label that a food has 20% of the DV of vitamin A, it means it has 20% of 900 mcg RAE, or 180 mcg RAE.

Because vitamin A is fat-soluble, it can accumulate in the liver. Over long-term high intakes, it can cause liver damage, dizziness, nausea, headaches, skin irritation, pain in joints, increased risk of fracture, and even coma and death.

Preformed vitamin A from animal foods or supplements can lead to these serious effects, but beta-carotene and other provitamin A carotenoids from plant foods is highly unlikely.

Preformed Vitamin A Upper Limit

AGE	AMOUNT
0–3 years	600 mcg RAE (2,000 IU)
4–8 years	900 mcg RAE (3,000 IU)
9–13 years	1,700 mcg RAE (5,667 IU)
14–18 years	2,800 mcg RAE (9,333 IU)
19+ years	3,000 mcg RAE (10,000 IU)
Pregnant or lactating: defer to upper limit by age	

Source: Institute of Medicine, Food and Nutrition Board, Dietary Reference Intakes

LUTEIN AND ZEAXANTHIN

Lutein and zeaxanthin are discussed together because they are usually found together and measured together in scientific studies. They are the two antioxidant carotenoids that build up the most in eyes and the brain, and have long been associated with eye health and prevention of age-related macular degeneration (AMD), the leading cause of blindness. They filter harmful blue light from UV exposure, and computer screens (including digital devices) to protect eye cells and keep them healthy. A 2018 study found that higher lutein status was also linked to better cognitive health throughout a person's life span. The neuroprotective role of both lutein and zeaxanthin may be due to their antioxidant activity, anti-inflammatory properties, and function in stabilizing cell membranes. As for a link between these nutrients and telomeres, the first study showing that older adults with higher lutein and zeaxanthin levels had longer telomeres was published in 2014.

These fat-soluble antioxidants are responsible for the yellow and green colors of many healthy foods including green vegetables, pistachios, avocados, and egg yolks. Pistachios, avocados, and eggs naturally contain fat, which helps the body absorb lutein and zeaxanthin. However, green vegetables don't and thus should be eaten in combination with a healthy fat to help with absorption. Olive oil, avocados, nuts, and seeds are all good sources of healthy fats that can be combined with green vegetables to enhance nutrient absorption. Other food sources include corn, kiwi, red grapes, zucchini, pumpkin, spinach, orange bell pepper, yellow squash, cucumber, peas parsley, and paprika. Our bodies do not make lutein and zeaxanthin, which is why it's important to find food sources.

Most green vegetables will lose a little lutein and zeaxanthin with cooking, but in some cases, amounts increase. This is true for mustard greens; these carotenoids more than double, from 3.7 mg to 10.4 mg per 3 to 4 ounces. For squash, they increase by nearly 70%, from 2.4 mg to 4.1 mg per cup. With collards, they go up by about 45%, from 4.3 mg to 6.2 mg per 3 to 4 ounces. At this time, there are no official recommended amounts of lutein and zeaxanthin for either foods or supplements, so the best advice is to eat a wide variety of naturally yellow and green foods, especially dark leafy greens. Getting a variety of lutein and zeaxanthin foods should get your intake up to or above what's been used in several studies (approximately 10 mg per day), without having to do any number crunching.

A Daily Value for lutein does not currently exist, although there is a strong interest in and a rationale for developing them. Americans average 1 to 2 mg per day. For now, the best estimate we have from the body of scientific literature is that 6 mg per day may be an effective level of lutein to reduce the risk of AMD. Lutein is likely safe at long-term doses up to 20 mg per day. Longer-term studies demonstrating the safety of doses are needed, although the daily intake from average food consumption is generally safe.

You can get your lutein level measured through a noninvasive eye test of macular pigment optical density (MPOD). Increased lutein intake can improve MPOD in about three months, even though it's normal for elevated serum levels to plateau after three weeks. Free lutein is more bioavailable than esterified lutein. Both forms exist in food and supplements, but naturally occurring lutein is primarily the more bioavailable free type. Esterified lutein is also absorbed but requires an additional step to be converted to free lutein, possibly affecting its absorption.

VITAMIN B12

Vitamin B12 is essential to the process that lowers levels of homocysteine (associated with heart disease) in the body. Dietary intake and blood levels of vitamin B12 have not been directly linked to telomere length. However, research has shown that women who take vitamin B12 supplements have longer telomeres compared with those who don't. We don't fully understand the mechanism behind this, but there are a few things that could be going on.

Vitamin B12 helps reduce oxidative stress by protecting glutathione, an important antioxidant found in our cells. (By the way, taking glutathione as a supplement has not been shown to increase glutathione levels in the body, but eating sulfurous foods like garlic, broccoli, asparagus, and avocados can lead to boosted levels.) Taking higher than needed levels of vitamin B12 may also reduce inflammation. These plausible mechanisms may explain why vitamin B12 supplement takers have longer telomeres, although more research is needed to confirm the hypothesis.

There's no upper limit set for vitamin B12 because the risk of toxicity is low. Vitamin B12 is a water-soluble vitamin bound to protein. The acidic environment in the stomach helps free vitamin B12 from protein so that it is available to combine with a compound called intrinsic factor (IF) in the small intestine. This new B12-IF package can be absorbed in the final part of the small intestine. The DV will be 2.4 mcg starting January 1, 2020. Individual needs may vary as noted in the table below.

Vitamin B12 Adequate Intake

AGE	AMOUNT
Birth to 6 months	0.4 mcg
7–12 months	0.5 mcg
1–3 years	0.9 mcg
4–8 years	1.2 mcg
9–13 years	1.8 mcg
14+	2.4 mcg
Pregnant	2.6 mcg
Lactating	2.8 mcg

Source: Institute of Medicine, Food and Nutrition Board, Dietary Reference Intakes

The supplemental form of vitamin B12 is already in the free form and doesn't need to go through the step of being separated from a protein. This is helpful when stomach acid or IF levels decline, which is common as we age. It is also useful for people who prefer not to eat foods from animal sources, which are natural sources of vitamin B12. In healthy adults, a little more than half of vitamin B12 (56%) is absorbed when the dose is 1 mcg. Absorption rates decline when IF is maxed out, which happens around 1 to 2 mcg. This is a good reason to include foods with vitamin B12 throughout the day.

Vitamin B12 Food Sources

FOOD	AMOUNT	% DV*
Clams, 3 ounces cooked	84 mcg	3,500%
Nutritional yeast, fortified, 1 tablespoon	6 mcg	250%
Rainbow trout, wild, 3 ounces cooked	5.4 mcg	225%
Salmon, 3 ounces cooked	4.8 mcg	200%
Rainbow trout, farmed, 3 ounces cooked	3.5 mcg	146%
Cereal, fortified, ¾ cup	2.9 mcg	121%
Tuna, light, canned, 3 ounces	2.5 mcg	104%
Haddock, 3 ounces cooked	1.8 mcg	75%
Milk, low-fat, 1 cup	1.2 mcg	50%
Egg, 1 large hard-boiled	0.6 mcg	25%
Chicken breast, 3 ounces cooked	0.3 mcg	13%

Source: USDA National Nutrient Database for Standard Reference Legacy Release

*The Daily Value (DV) used for these calculations is 2.4 mcg per the 2020–2021 labeling update.

FOLATE

Folate is a B vitamin with an important role in maintaining the integrity of DNA and DNA methylation (a simple and common transfer of a methyl group from one molecule to another occurring in healthy bodies all the time). Methylation can only work well if there's enough folate in the diet from natural foods, fortified foods, or supplements (the supplement form of folate is folic acid). Folate helps generate a universal methyl donor called s-adenosyl methionine (SAM), which is used throughout the body.

Some studies have shown that blood levels of folate are associated with telomere length in both men and women. Low folate can lead to telomere DNA damage. This may be why poor folate intake is associated with shorter telomeres. It appears that low folate status also leads to imbalances that shorten telomeres.

Paradoxically, very poor DNA methylation can lead to longer than normal telomeres. Longer telomeres were seen in men with very low folate status, but not in women with a similar status. The exact reasons for the difference are not known.

Because there are different forms of folate with different biological potency, the recommendations are described in micrograms of dietary folate equivalents, or DFEs: 1 mcg folate from food is the same as 1 mcg DFE, which is equivalent to 0.5 mcg (on an empty stomach) and 0.6 mcg (with food) folic acid. Folic acid is more bioavailable, so less is needed. The DV on nutrition labels is 400 mcg, but needs may be higher or lower depending on age.

Dietary Folate Recommendations per Day

AGE	DIETARY FOLATE EQUIVALENTS (DFE)
Birth to 6 months	65 mcg
7–12 months	80 mcg
1–3 years	150 mcg
4–8 years	200 mcg
9–13 years	300 mcg
14–18 years	400 mcg
19+ years	400 mcg
Pregnant or lactating: defer to upper limit by age	

Source: Institute of Medicine, Food and Nutrition Board, Dietary Reference Intakes

Folate is found in vegetables, fruits, nuts, beans, peas, seafood, eggs, dairy products, meat, poultry, and whole grains. In the United States and Canada, because refined grains are so widely consumed, many products made from grains, such as cereals, are fortified with folic acid to reduce the risk of neural tube defects. Other reasons to appreciate folate: having normal folate levels may lower the risk for depression, may improve the response to antidepressants for people who do suffer from depression, and is naturally found in foods associated with a lower risk of cancers and heart disease.

According to data from the 2013–2014 NHANES, most Americans are getting adequate folate. However, among females ages 14 to 30 and black women, about one in five aren't meeting their daily requirements. Other groups that may be at risk are alcoholics, pregnant and lactating women, people with malabsorption conditions such as celiac disease or inflammatory bowel disease, and individuals with a genetic impairment that limits the conversion of folate to its biologically active form.

Taking too much folic acid also carries risks. In older adults, it may mask a vitamin B12 deficiency, which can cause irreversible neurological damage. There are also concerns that very high intakes could spur the development of early lesions that increase the risk of certain cancers. Mothers who took 1,000 mcg or more per day around the conception period saw lower cognitive development scores in their children at 4 to 5 years of age compared with mothers who took 400 to 999 mcg. Further, when there is excessive folic acid in the body, some is left unmetabolized, which has been linked to fewer and less active immune system fighter cells. Therefore, the upper limit of folic acid is 800 mcg for pregnant or lactating adults. This is for the supplemental form only, so there's no reason to convert it to a measure that is comparable to food sources of folate (but if you'd like to know, it's 1,666 DFE).

Supplemental Folic Acid Upper Limit

AGE	AMOUNT
Birth to 6 months	n/a*
7–12 months	n/a*
1–3 years	300 mcg
4–8 years	400 mcg
9–13 years	600 mcg
14–18 years	800 mcg
19+ years	1,000 mcg
Pregnant or lactating: defer to upper limit by age	

Source: Institute of Medicine, Food and Nutrition Board, Dietary Reference Intakes

*Breast milk, formula, and food should be the only sources of folate from 0–12 months.

There is no upper limit for folate from food. Food sources of folate have not been known to cause any of the issues seen with supplemental folic acid. Depending on your individual needs, a combination of food and supplement may be right for you. However, it's important to remember that food sources of folate are a safer choice and offer additional nourishment. For example, leafy greens offer many vitamins, minerals, polyphenols, and fiber; they're not simply a source of folate.

Anything with 10% or more of the DV for folate is a good source of the nutrient, but even including foods with lower levels contributes to your overall intake. In the table on page 65 are just a few examples of some healthy foods that provide folate along with additional nourishment, whether it's fiber, plant protein, antioxidants, essential minerals, or other phytonutrients.

Folate Food Sources

FOOD	AMOUNT	% DV*
Spinach, ½ cup cooked	131 mcg	33%
Black-eyed peas, ½ cup cooked	105 mcg	26%
Asparagus, 4 spears boiled	89 mcg	22%
Brussels sprouts, ½ cup cooked	78 mcg	20%
Romaine lettuce, 1 cup	64 mcg	16%
Avocado, ½ cup	59 mcg	15%
Spinach, 1 cup raw	58 mcg	15%
Broccoli, ½ cup cooked	52 mcg	13%
Mustard greens, ½ cup cooked	52 mcg	13%
Green peas, ½ cup cooked	47 mcg	12%
Kidney beans, canned, ½ cup cooked	46 mcg	12%
Wheat germ, 2 tablespoons	40 mcg	10%
Turnip greens, ½ cup cooked	32 mcg	8%
Orange, 1 small	29 mcg	7%
Papaya, ½ cup	27 mcg	7%
Banana, 1 medium	24 mcg	6%
Egg, 1 large, hard-boiled	22 mcg	6%

Source: USDA National Nutrient Database for Standard Reference Legacy Release
*The Daily Value (DV) used for these calculations is 400 mcg DFE.

VITAMIN C

Vitamin C, a powerful antioxidant found in many fruits and vegetables, which are the foundation of every healthy diet. Animal studies show that vitamin C stops telomere shortening, extends life span, and fights oxidative stress and excessive release of inflammatory compounds. These animal studies also show the potential role of vitamin C, as part of a healthy diet in preventing Alzheimer's disease, perhaps by trapping free radicals, suppressing pro-inflammatory genes, alleviating neuroinflammation, and curbing the formation of amyloid-beta tangles in the brain, a hallmark of Alzheimer's.

The natural form of vitamin C is called ascorbate, and the synthetic form is called ascorbic acid. Research suggests that there isn't a significant difference in their bioavailability to the body. Nevertheless, keep in mind that fruits and vegetables containing vitamin C have the benefit of providing a variety of other healthful nutrients and phytochemicals. The DV will be 90 mg starting January 1, 2020.

Vitamin C Recommendations per Day

AGE	MALE	FEMALE
0–6 months	40 mg	40 mg
0–12 months	50 mg	50 mg
1–3 years	15 mg	15 mg
4–8 years	25 mg	25 mg
9–13 years	45 mg	45 mg
14–18 years	75 mg	65 mg 80 mg (pregnant) 115 mg (lactating)
19+ years	90 mg	75 mg 85 mg (pregnant) 120 mg (lactating)
Smokers: add 35 mg/day		

Source: Institute of Medicine, Food and Nutrition Board, Dietary Reference Intakes

Vitamin C Food Sources

FOOD	AMOUNT	% DV*
Sweet red pepper, fresh, ½ cup	95 mg	106%
Orange, medium	70 mg	78%
Kiwifruit, medium	64 mg	71%
Broccoli, ½ cup cooked	51 mg	57%
Strawberries, sliced, ½ cup	49 mg	54%
Brussels sprouts, ½ cup cooked	48 mg	53%
Cantaloupe, ½ cup	29 mg	32%
Baked potato, medium	17 mg	19%
Tomato, medium, fresh	17 mg	19%
Spinach, ½ cup cooked	9 mg	10%
Green peas, ½ cup cooked from frozen	8 mg	9%

Source: USDA National Nutrient Database for Standard Reference Legacy Release

*The Daily Value (DV) used for these calculations is 90 mg per the 2020–2021 labeling update.

The risk of long-term excessive vitamin C from food is low. Getting too much from supplements can lead to diarrhea, nausea, abdominal cramps, and other gastrointestinal distress. These problems are caused by unabsorbed vitamin C in the digestive tract.

Supplemental Vitamin C Upper Limit

AGE	AMOUNT
0–12 months	not established
1–3 years	400 mg
4–8 years	650 mg
9–13 years	1,200 mg
14–18 years	1,800 mg
19+ years	2,000 mg
Pregnant or lactating: defer to upper limit by age	

Source: Institute of Medicine, Food and Nutrition Board, Dietary Reference Intakes

VITAMIN D

Missing out on vitamin D can mean shorter telomeres and genomic instability, according to a nationally representative study of Americans ages 40 to 59 years. In this study, 20 ng/mL of circulating vitamin D as measured by blood test, was considered optimal. Your physician can run this test for you and may recommend supplemental vitamin D until your levels stabilize. Once your vitamin D is where it should be, the daily recommended amount is 20 mcg for most people (ages 14 to 70 years). In the first year of life, the recommendation is 400 IU (10 mcg), and after age 70, the recommended intake gets bumped up to 800 IU (20 mcg).

Most Americans are not getting enough vitamin D, which is a public health concern because low intakes are linked to all-cause mortality and cancer. Our bodies can produce vitamin D with sun exposure, which is not possible in all seasons in all geographical areas. Other sources include a limited number of natural foods, fortified foods, and supplements.

The best food sources of vitamin D are fatty fish such as salmon, tuna, and sardines. Smaller amounts of vitamin D are found in egg yolks—one more reason to eat the whole egg. For a plant-based option, some mushrooms exposed to UV light under controlled conditions provide up to 100% DV and will be specially labeled as such. Like us, these special mushrooms can convert ultraviolet (UV) light into vitamin D.

Fortified foods (milk, ready-to-eat cereal, and some brands of orange juice and yogurt) are another option to increase vitamin D intake. Check the label for the amount of vitamin D in a product.

VITAMIN D WILL SOON
BE EASIER TO FIND

As of 2020, when nutrition labels are changing, for the first time vitamin D will be listed on all labels as a required nutrient. This will make it much easier for us to understand how much of this important nutrient our food choices contain. Large food makers have until New Year's Day 2020 to make the updates (smaller food companies have an extra year to comply). The DV will be 20 mcg.

Vitamin D Recommendations

AGE	PER DAY
0–12 months	10 mcg
1–70 years	15 mcg
71+ years	20 mcg
Pregnant or lactating: defer to upper limit by age	

Source: Institute of Medicine, Food and Nutrition Board, Dietary Reference Intakes

Vitamin D Food Sources

FOOD	AMOUNT	% DV*
Mushrooms, fortified, 2–3 ounces raw	20 mcg	100%
Salmon, 3 ounces cooked	11 mcg	55%
Milk, fortified, 8 ounces	3.2 mcg	16%
Orange juice, fortified, 8 ounces	2.5 mcg	13%
Yogurt, fortified, 6 ounces	2 mcg	10%
Cereal, fortified, ¾–1 cup	2 mcg	10%
Tuna, canned in water, 3 ounces	1.7 mcg	9%
Sardines, canned in oil, 2 medium	1.2 mcg	6%
Egg, 1 large	1 mcg	5%

Source: USDA National Nutrient Database for Standard Reference Legacy Release

*The Daily Value (DV) used for these calculations is 20 mcg per the 2020–2021 labeling update.

Excessive vitamin D is not possible from sun exposure. It is also unlikely from food sources. However, supplemental vitamin D doses may be high enough to exceed the recommended upper limit. Long-term high intakes can damage the heart, blood vessels, and kidneys.

Supplemental Vitamin D Upper Limit

AGE	PER DAY
0–6 months	25 mcg
7–12 months	38 mcg
1–3 years	63 mcg
4–8 years	75 mcg
9+ years	100 mcg
Pregnant or lactating: defer to upper limit by age	

Source: Institute of Medicine, Food and Nutrition Board, Dietary Reference Intakes

VITAMIN E

Vitamin E from either food or supplements is associated with longer telomeres. In women, research suggests a dose-dependent relationship, meaning the more vitamin E, the longer the telomeres. Vitamin E is a well-known antioxidant that may help to alleviate the effects of oxidative stress. It is commonly found in extra-virgin olive oil and nuts. The DV will be 15 mg starting January 1, 2020.

Recommended Vitamin E

AGE	PER DAY
0–6 months	4 mg
7–12 months	5 mg
1–3 years	6 mg
4–8 years	7 mg
9–13 years	11 mg
14+ years	15 mg
Pregnant or lactating: 15 mg	

Source: Institute of Medicine, Food and Nutrition Board, Dietary Reference Intakes

Vitamin E Food Sources

FOOD	AMOUNT	% DV*
Sunflower seeds, 1 ounce	7.4 mg	49%
Almonds, 1 ounce	6.8 mg	45%
Sunflower oil, 1 tablespoon	5.6 mg	37%
Safflower oil, 1 tablespoon	4.6 mg	31%
Hazelnuts, 1 ounce	4.3 mg	29%
Peanut butter, 2 tablespoons	2.9 mg	19%
Spinach, ½ cup cooked	1.2 mg	8%
Kiwifruit, medium	1.1 mg	7%
Mango, sliced, ½ cup	0.7 mg	5%
Tomato, medium	0.7 mg	5%
Spinach, 1 cup raw	0.6 mg	4%

Source: USDA National Nutrient Database for Standard Reference Legacy Release

*The DV used for these calculations is 15 mg per the 2020–2021 labeling update.

There are no negative effects from consuming vitamin E in food, but high doses from supplements may increase the risk of hemorrhagic stroke.

Supplemental Vitamin E Upper Limit

AGE	PER DAY
1–3 years	200 mg
4–8 years	300 mg
9–13 years	600 mg
14–18 years	800 mg
19+ years	1,000 mg
Pregnant or lactating: defer to upper limit by age	

Source: Institute of Medicine, Food and Nutrition Board, Dietary Reference Intakes

COPPER

Copper is an essential trace mineral whose intake was associated with longer telomeres in a recent analysis of data from more than 7,000 U.S. adults. Prior to this study, copper's relationship to telomere length had not been well studied.

The researchers found that women had longer telomeres than men, a result seen in other studies. They also found that obesity did not impact the effect of copper. This was surprising as they had hypothesized that a high BMI, shown to negatively impact telomere length, could overpower the results for copper. They found minor differences, but not enough to discount the unique role of copper in telomere health.

The fact that copper is a major component of a group of enzymes called superoxide dismutases (SODs), the body's self-made antioxidants, may account for its importance in telomere health. SODs, which disarm DNA-damaging free radicals, are present inside cells, inside mitochondria, and outside cells. Copper and zinc are major components in two of the three forms of SODs.

Copper is needed in small amounts and is found in many foods such as oysters and other shellfish, whole grains, beans, nuts, and potatoes. Smaller but still significant amounts are found in dark leafy green vegetables such as kale and broccoli as well as in dried fruit, cocoa, dark chocolate, and black pepper. Copper works with iron to form red blood cells and helps with iron absorption.

It is possible to take in too much copper, which can be poisonous, so note the upper limit as well as recommended intake levels. The DV will be 0.9 mg starting January 1, 2020.

Recommended Copper

AGE	PER DAY
Birth to 6 months	.2 mg
7–12 months	.22 mg
1–3 years	.34 mg
4–8 years	.44 mg
9–13 years	.7 mg
14–18 years	.89 mg
19+ years	.9 mg
Pregnant: 1 mg; lactating: 1.3 mg	

Source: Institute of Medicine, Food and Nutrition Board, Dietary Reference Intakes

Copper Upper Limit

AGE	PER DAY
Birth to 6 months	not established
7–12 months	not established
1–3 years	1 mg
4–8 years	3 mg
9–13 years	5 mg
14–18 years	8 mg
19+ years	10 mg
Pregnant or lactating: defer to upper limit by age	

Source: Institute of Medicine, Food and Nutrition Board, Dietary Reference Intakes

Copper Food Sources

FOOD	AMOUNT	% DV
Oysters, 3 ounces cooked	4.9 mg	544%
Cashews, dry roasted, ¼ cup	0.8 mg	89%
Sunflower seeds, toasted, ¼ cup	0.6 mg	67%
Hazelnuts, ¼ cup	0.5 mg	55%
Tofu, firm, ½ cup	0.5 mg	55%
Walnuts, ¼ cup	0.5 mg	55%
Spirulina dried seaweed, 1 tablespoon	0.4 mg	44%
Pistachios, dry roasted, ¼ cup	0.4 mg	44%
Almonds, dry roasted, ¼ cup	0.4 mg	44%
Sesame seeds, 1 tablespoon	0.4 mg	44%
Red kidney beans, canned, ½ cup	0.4 mg	44%
Tomato puree, canned, ½ cup	0.4 mg	40%
Cocoa, 1 tablespoon	0.2 mg	22%
Prunes, ¼ cup	0.2 mg	22%
White mushrooms, ¼ cup cooked	0.2 mg	22%
Sun-dried tomatoes, ¼ cup	0.2 mg	22%
Apricots, dried, ¼ cup	0.2 mg	22%

Source: USDA National Nutrient Database for Standard Reference Legacy Release

*The Daily Value (DV) used for these calculations is 0.9 mg per the 2020–2021 labeling update.

MAGNESIUM

In animal and cell studies, long-term magnesium deficiency has been associated with shorter telomeres and increased oxidative stress, a known contributor to telomere deterioration. Human studies have shown links between dietary magnesium and longer telomeres in women, and between low levels of circulating magnesium and high levels of inflammatory markers. When the body does not have enough magnesium, its DNA-repairing capability declines and abnormalities in chromosomes can form. Low magnesium may influence telomere health through increases in oxidative stress and inflammation as well as a weakening of DNA integrity.

The majority of Americans are not getting enough magnesium through food, but supplements seem to compensate for any deficiency. The DV will be 420 mg starting January 1, 2020.

Magnesium Recommendations per Day

AGE	MALE	FEMALE
0–6 months	30 mg	30 mg
7–12 months	75 mg	75 mg
1–3 years	80 mg	80 mg
4–8 years	130 mg	130 mg
9–13 years	240 mg	240 mg
14–18 years	410 mg	360 mg 400 mg (pregnant) 360 mg (lactating)
19–30 years	400 mg	310 mg 350 mg (pregnant) 310 mg (lactating)
31–50 years+	420 mg	320 mg 360 mg (pregnant) 320 mg (lactating)

Source: Institute of Medicine, Food and Nutrition Board, Dietary Reference Intakes

Magnesium Food Sources

FOOD	AMOUNT	% DV
Almonds, 1 ounce	80 mg	19%
Spinach, ½ cup cooked	78 mg	19%
Cashews, 1 ounce	74 mg	18%
Peanuts, ¼ cup	63 mg	15%
Soymilk, 8 ounces	61 mg	15%
Black beans, ½ cup cooked	60 mg	14%
Edamame, shelled, ½ cup cooked	50 mg	12%
Whole wheat bread, 2 slices	46 mg	11%
Avocado, 1 cup	44 mg	10%
Brown rice, ½ cup cooked	42 mg	10%
Salmon, 3 ounces cooked	26 mg	6%
Halibut, 3 ounces cooked	24 mg	6%

Source: USDA National Nutrient Database for Standard Reference Legacy Release

*The Daily Value (DV) used for these calculations is 420 mg per the 2020–2021 labeling update.

Getting too much magnesium from food sources isn't a concern for healthy people with working kidneys who are able to remove any excess magnesium in urine. High doses from supplements can lead to diarrhea, nausea, and abdominal cramps, and very large doses can be fatal.

Supplemental Magnesium Upper Limit

AGE	MALE	FEMALE
0–12 months	Not established	Not established
1–3 years	65 mg	65 mg
4–8 years	110 mg	110 mg
9+ years	350 mg	350 mg
Pregnant or lactating: defer to upper limit by age		

Source: Institute of Medicine, Food and Nutrition Board, Dietary Reference Intakes

ZINC

In cell studies, adding zinc promoted the activity of telomerase, the telomere-lengthening enzyme that adds bits of DNA back on telomeres. Although the exact mechanism of zinc in telomere health for humans is not exactly understood, human studies have demonstrated that zinc deficiency can cause DNA damage. Research shows that low zinc is associated with oxidative damage and that zinc supplements can reduce oxidative stress and inflammation. Zinc also decreases the rate of infection, another known cause of telomere shortening.

Most children and adults in the United States get enough zinc. However, 35% to 45% of adults 60 years and older do not get the recommended amount. The DV will be 11 mg starting January 1, 2020.

Zinc Recommendations per Day

AGE	MALE	FEMALE
0–6 months	2 mg	40 mg
7–12 months	3 mg	50 mg
1–3 years	3 mg	15 mg
4–8 years	5 mg	25 mg
9–13 years	8 mg	45 mg
14–18 years	11 mg	9 mg 12 mg (pregnant) 13 mg (lactating)
19+ years	11 mg	8 mg 11 mg (pregnant) 12 mg (lactating)

Source: Institute of Medicine, Food and Nutrition Board, Dietary Reference Intakes

Zinc Food Sources

FOOD	ZINC	% DV
Oysters, 3 ounces cooked	74 mg	673%
Alaskan king crab, 3 ounces cooked	6.5 mg	59%
Cereal, fortified, ¾ cup	3.8 mg	35%
Lobster, 3 ounces cooked	3.4 mg	31%
Pumpkin seeds, dried, 1 ounce	2.2 mg	20%
Cashews, 1 ounce	1.6 mg	15%
Chickpeas, ½ cup cooked	1.3 mg	12%
Instant oatmeal, 1 packet with water	1.1 mg	10%
Almonds, 1 ounce	0.9 mg	8%
Boneless, skinless chicken breast, 3 ounces cooked	0.9 mg	8%

Source: USDA National Nutrient Database for Standard Reference Legacy Release

*The Daily Value (DV) used for these calculations is 11 mg per the 2020–2021 labeling update.

Short- and long-term overdoses of zinc have consequences. Excessive amounts in the short term can cause nausea, vomiting, loss of appetite, abdominal cramps, diarrhea, and headaches. Long-term high intakes result in a depressed immune system and disruption of the urinary system and metabolism of some essential minerals such as iron and copper.

Zinc Upper Limit

AGE	AMOUNT
0–6 months	4 mg
7–12 months	5 mg
1–3 years	7 mg
4–8 years	12 mg
9–13 years	23 mg
14–18 years	34 mg
19+ years	40 mg
Pregnant or lactating: defer to upper limit by age	

Source: Institute of Medicine, Food and Nutrition Board, Dietary Reference Intakes

FIBER

For each gram of fiber you eat per 1,000 calories, you could earn about eight more base pairs on your telomeres, according to the nationwide NHANES study. It found a dose-dependent relationship between fiber and telomeres. That means as consumption of fiber increases, so does telomere length.

NHANES found a cellular aging benefit at 10 grams of fiber per 1,000 calories (that's 20 grams of fiber for someone who consumes 2,000 calories daily). Regular consumption of that amount of fiber could take 4.8 years off a person's biological age. This is a lower level than the 14 grams per 1,000 calories recommended by the Dietary Guidelines for Americans. However, the linear relationship between fiber and telomere length suggests that even if you can get the biological aging benefits of fiber intake at the level noted by NHANES, there are likely benefits at higher levels, such as those set by the Dietary Guidelines.

Unfortunately, the same study found that American adults get an average of less than 16 grams of fiber a day. At the same time that the majority of Americans are not meeting the goal for fiber intake, new recommendations are increasing the goal amount. In a 2016 update from the FDA, the DV (used in food labeling) for dietary fiber was increased from 25 grams to 28 grams a day per 2,000 calories. Remember, this is a general number, but estimated individual daily minimums could vary from as little as 19 grams for toddlers to 38 grams for men in their teens through their forties. Generally, there's no upper limit on fiber, and its bulky nature is self-limiting. That said, it's best to increase your daily fiber intake gradually if you're concerned about gastrointestinal side effects such as gas or bloating. Food sources (fruits, vegetables, whole grains, beans, and nuts) are gentler on the stomach than synthetic or isolated supplement forms.

While scientists don't know exactly how fiber keeps telomeres longer, there are a couple of possible reasons. One, there is good evidence that telomere length and biological aging are closely linked to inflammation and oxidative stress. Many studies show that as dietary fiber intake increases, markers for inflammation and oxidative stress decline, even after adjusting for demographic and lifestyle factors. Two, fiber moderates blood sugar spikes, and we know that as blood glucose rises so do inflammation and oxidative stress. Because fiber slows down sugar absorption, it helps lower blood glucose levels and insulin resistance, decreasing the risk for developing type 2 diabetes.

The bottom line: Not eating enough dietary fiber can increase the risk of accelerated aging. People who ate the least fiber per day were five to six years biologically older than those who ate the most. Telomere health research supports 28 grams of fiber a day or more. Dietary fiber is found in most plant foods such as fruits, vegetables, whole grains, beans, and nuts.

OMEGA-3s

Many research studies have already shown us that omega-3 fatty acids from marine sources (fish and seaweed) help people with heart disease live longer. A recent study suggests that telomere length may be one of the mechanisms behind the benefit, and omega-3s may protect telomeres by reducing oxidative stress and inflammation.

Five years of data from more than 600 stable heart disease patients indicated that the more marine-based omega-3s the patients had circulating in their blood, the longer their telomeres. The specific types of omega-3s were eicosapentaenoic acid (EPA) and docosahexaenoic acid (DHA). The relationship was linear, which means that the more omega-3s, the greater the telomere protection. These fats might work by dampening inflammation-promoting molecules (also known as proinflammatory cytokines). Indeed, the more omega-3s in the blood, the less inflammatory chemical production.

In a four-month randomized controlled trial, a daily dose of 1.25 grams of omega-3s decreased an inflammatory marker called interleukin 6 (IL-6) by 10%. A higher dose of 2.5 grams per day dampened IL-6 by even more: 12%. Meanwhile, the control group experienced a 36% increase in IL-6.

To reduce deaths from heart disease and to support healthy pregnancy outcomes, the American Heart Association and the Dietary Guidelines for Americans recommend consuming 8 ounces of seafood a week to get an average of 250 to 500 mg EPA+DHA a day. People with heart disease should aim for 1,000 mg a day. The simple take-home message is to enjoy a 4-ounce serving of seafood twice a week.

Seafood by Omega-3 Content
(per 4 ounces cooked)

1,000+ MG	500–999 MG	250–499 MG	LESS THAN 250 MG
Anchovies*	Albacore tuna	Catfish*	Cod*
Herring*	Alaskan pollock*	Clams*	Crayfish*
Mackerel (Atlantic and Pacific)*	Barramundi*	Flounder/sole*	Haddock*
Sablefish (black cod)	Crab*	Grouper	Lobster*
Salmon (Atlantic, Chinook, coho)*	Mussels*	Halibut	Mahi mahi
Swordfish^	Salmon (chum, pink, sockeye)*	King mackerel^	Shrimp*
Trout*	Sea bass	Perch*	Scallops*
	Squid*	Rockfish	Tilapia*
	Tilefish^	Skipjack tuna (common "light" canned tuna)*	Yellowfin tuna
	Walleye	Snapper	

*lower in mercury   ^higher in mercury

MERCURY IN SEAFOOD

Worries over mercury should be weighed against the risks of not consuming enough seafood. In addition to potentially lengthening telomeres, seafood provides the omega-3s the brain needs to develop and function optimally. Maternal fish intake has even been shown to boost the baby's IQ by an average of 5.8 points. People who eat fish are 20% less likely to be depressed. Eating seafood at least twice a week reduces the risk of death by 17%.

The FDA and Environmental Protection Agency (EPA) allow for a 1,000% uncertainty factor when setting mercury limits on seafood, and still you could eat more than 100 pounds of shrimp per week before there was a risk. About 90% of the seafood Americans eat is low in mercury. To provide a few more examples, the upper limit for salmon is more than 50 pounds a week; for tilapia it's more than 90 pounds. You could still eat 3.5 pounds a week of albacore tuna, a fish that is relatively high in mercury compared to lower-mercury choices. But most Americans don't even get the 8 ounces a week recommended by the Dietary Guidelines for Americans, American Heart Association, American Diabetes Association, American Pediatric Association, National Alzheimer's Association, American Psychiatric Association, and other organizations.

Plant Sources of Omega-3s

Some very healthy plant foods—including chia seeds, walnuts, flaxseeds, soy foods, and leafy greens—provide a different kind of omega-3 fat called ALA. Only about 1% is converted to EPA+DHA, but there are plenty of other health benefits to foods high in ALA such as their anti-inflammatory and antioxidant properties. Typically, people get enough ALA through food.

Omega-3 Supplements

Supplements should be used in addition to a healthy diet, not in place of one. They should only be used when they are needed to fill a gap that you can't meet through your diet. Food sources have many more benefits than supplements: they decrease the risk of taking excessive amounts of a nutrient and also come in a package of other nutrients. For example, salmon doesn't just supply anti-inflammatory omega-3s. It also provides lean protein, hard-to-get vitamin D, B vitamins, brain-healthy choline, and antioxidants—and can be part of a delicious meal. That said, sometimes supplements are helpful, depending on your individual need. Brands such as Nordic Naturals and Carlson promise a level of quality assurance in the amount of omega-3s they contain, freshness, and testing for contaminants. The bottom line: Choose food first and supplements when advised.

FAT FACTS

Dietary fat can be confusing, so here's a quick primer. Generally, fat is categorized as saturated or unsaturated. The more unsaturated it is, the healthier it tends to be. This is really what it comes down to, but continue to read if you're curious about the chemistry.

The saturated/unsaturated designation is based on the number of double bonds a fat molecule has. Saturated fatty acid, or SAFA, is completely saturated and has no double bonds. It's more or less solid at room temperature. Think of butter and coconut oil. Unsaturated fats have one or more double bonds. If it's only one, it's called a monounsaturated fatty acid, or MUFA. If there's more than one double bond, it's called a polyunsaturated fatty acid, or PUFA. Both MUFAs and PUFAs tend to be liquid at room temperature. Think of olive oil, grapeseed oil, and canola oil. However, some MUFAs and PUFAs are found in foods that seem solid, such as salmon, walnuts, and pistachios.

If you're still following, it gets more complicated. Many of the fats we eat are actually a blend of types of fats. For example, olive oil has SAFA, MUFA and PUFA, although it's mostly MUFA. One PUFA that we've been discussing are omega-3s. You've already read about three kinds of omega-3s (EPA, DHA, and ALA). There is some research suggesting that the more omega-3 than omega-6 you consume, the better. That's because omega-3s tend to cool inflammation, and omega-6s tend to flame it. This relationship is known as the omega-6:omega-3 ratio. Given that most people don't get enough omega-3s, any increase will likely shift this ratio in the right direction.

If you're confused, you're not alone. There is much more to the world of dietary fats, and you don't need to know it all. The big picture takeaway is to get more unsaturated fats than saturated ones.

CURCUMIN

Curcumin, a component of turmeric, may have an interesting role in shortening telomeres and inhibiting telomerase in cancer cells without damaging normal cells. In a study of brain tumor cells, researchers found that curcumin bound to cells that showed telomerase activity, such as cancer cells. It infiltrated and initiated cell death.

A polyphenol widely used in Ayurvedic medicine, curcumin is being studied for its antioxidant and anti-inflammatory benefits. More research is needed to confirm its benefits, but in the meantime the research results are fascinating.

In other good news, curcumin immediately improved working memory and prolonged focus in a randomized double-blind placebo-controlled clinical trial with a healthy elderly population. With regular use over a four-week span, curcumin also led to less fatigue and better mood. For this short-term experiment, the participants consumed 400 mg of a curcumin supplement, then their attention and memory were tested one hour later and again three hours later.

Curcumin is a root that looks like an orange version of ginger. In fact, curcumin and ginger are botanically related. Just as there are various forms of ginger—fresh, dried, candied, ground—there are multiple forms of turmeric, although it is most commonly found in the United States as a ground spice on its own or as part of curry powder.

A study of 28 spice products labeled either turmeric or curry powder found that pure turmeric powder contains an average of about 3% curcumin, whereas curry powders have a wide range of curcumin levels, all relatively low compared with turmeric. A tablespoon of turmeric is 6.8 grams, 3% (about 200 mg) of which is curcumin. It's safe in amounts normally found in foods, but long-term use at high doses (e.g., 2 grams or more) found in supplements may present issues. Be sure to discuss curcumin supplements with a qualified health provider before taking any.

The bad news is that curcumin is poorly absorbed, but there's an easy fix. A compound called piperine in black pepper increases the bioavailability of curcumin by 2,000%. The take-home message: Cook with both turmeric and black pepper for nutrient absorption and a great flavor combination.

POLYPHENOLS

Polyphenols are a large class of molecules found in many whole natural foods. They vary in their specific activities, but, in general, a diet high in polyphenols tends to improve telomere health. It also reduces oxidative stress and inflammation, improve the function of mitochondria (the organelles inside our cells that convert food to energy), and reduce amyloid plaque formation, one of the hallmarks of Alzheimer's disease.

Early exploration into the health benefits of polyphenols focused on their strong antioxidant properties, but current scientific research suggests that they are more than just antioxidants. They interact with the gut microbiome (the community of bacteria, generally nonpathogenic, in the gut), and the products of their metabolism influence how cells talk to each other in order to keep the body healthy.

Foods that are highest in polyphenols by weight include spices, fruit, seeds, vegetables, nonalcoholic beverages, whole grains, cacao foods, alcoholic beverages, and cooking oils such as extra-virgin olive oil. The "by weight" caveat is important because gram for gram, it's more likely you'll eat a heaping cup of broccoli (100 grams) than a cup of ground cloves (100 grams). So even though spices are a potent source of polyphenols, and make a great addition to healthy recipes, you'll get more total polyphenols from coffee or quinoa than a pinch of chile powder.

It is more useful to look at top sources of polyphenols by food group. Foods can really only be compared fairly if they were analyzed the same way, and there are a few different ways to measure. Following are examples of some of the top 100 polyphenol foods as measured by chromatography. Also keep in mind that if a food isn't listed (such as your favorite superhealthy vegetable, nut, or whole grain), don't dismiss it. Perhaps there simply isn't published data on its polyphenol content. The best and easiest way to ensure you're getting a good variety and amount of polyphenols is by incorporating foods from the high polyphenol food groups throughout the day (see the lists starting on page 88).

WHAT'S A POLYPHENOL?

Polyphenols are a class of chemical compound found in a wide variety of natural plant foods such as berries, broccoli, beans, onions, olive oil, red wine, citrus, cocoa, tea, coffee, spices, and other fruits and vegetables; they give many plants their color. Polyphenols have antioxidant activity, but recently researchers have been exploring their role in health beyond their antioxidant power. Polyphenols can act as antioxidants, are prebiotics (food for good bacteria in the gut), improve blood flow through blood vessel dilation, and adapt the body's immune response, although how exactly they do all of that is still under study.

In terms of chemistry, a polyphenol is any compound with a phenolic ring as part of its molecular structure, but the category is at least 8,000 types strong and very diverse with many subgroups. Flavonoids are one of the largest subgroups (more than 5,000 have been identified), and the flavonoid group can be broken down further into subtypes: flavonols, flavones, flavan-3-ols, flavanones, anthocyanidins, and isoflavones. There are five main subgroups within the nonflavonoid group: phenolic acids, lignans, stilbenes, tannins, and lignins. An amazing free online resource is the Phenol-Explorer (http://phenol-explorer.eu), which is the first comprehensive database on polyphenol content in foods, with more than 400 entries.

A number of cell studies reveal how polyphenols may be working to impact telomere health. Curcumin has been shown to slow the rate of telomere shortening and resveratrol to cause instability in the telomeres of cancer cells. The main point is that polyphenols are natural plant compounds found in a wide variety of wholesome foods known for antioxidant and anti-inflammatory characteristics, for support of mitochondrial health, and for telomere maintenance. Following are some common foods organized by categories and in order of the food's polyphenol rank.

Seasonings and Oils High in Polyphenols

1. Cloves
2. Peppermint, dried
3. Star anise
4. Mexican oregano, dried
5. Celery seed
6. Common sage, dried
7. Rosemary, dried
8. Spearmint, dried
9. Common thyme, dried
10. Capers
11. Sweet basil, dried
12. Curry powder
13. Ginger, dried
14. Common thyme, fresh
15. Lemon verbena, dried
16. Extra-virgin olive oil
17. Cumin
18. Chinese cinnamon
19. Caraway
20. Ceylon cinnamon
21. Parsley, dried
22. Marjoram, dried
23. Rapeseed oil
24. Vinegar

Fruits High in Polyphenols

1. Black chokeberry
2. Black elderberry
3. Lowbush blueberry
4. Black currant
5. Highbush blueberry
6. Plum
7. Sweet cherry
8. Blackberry
9. Strawberry
10. Red raspberry
11. Prune
12. Black grape
13. Apple
14. Peach
15. Red currant
16. Apricot
17. Nectarine
18. Quince
19. Pear
20. Green grape

Nuts, Seeds, and Beans High in Polyphenols

1. Soy cheese
2. Soybean sprout
3. Walnut
4. Soy tofu
5. White bean
6. Black bean
7. Soy meat
8. Soy yogurt
9. Tempeh (fermented soybeans)
10. Almond
11. Roasted soybean
12. Soy flour
13. Pecan
14. Hazelnut
15. Chestnut
16. Flaxseed meal

Vegetables High in Polyphenols

1. Black olive
2. Green olive
3. Globe artichoke head
4. Red chicory
5. Red onion
6. Green chicory
7. Spinach
8. Shallot
9. Yellow onion
10. Broccoli
11. Asparagus
12. Potato
13. Curly endive
14. Red lettuce
15. Endive (escarole)
16. Carrot

Nonalcoholic Beverages High in Polyphenols

1. Coffee, filtered
2. Black tea
3. Green tea
4. Unfiltered apple juice
5. 100% pomegranate juice
6. 100% blood orange juice
7. 100% grapefruit juice
8. 100% orange juice
9. 100% lemon juice
10. Chocolate milk
11. Soy milk
12. Pure pomelo juice

Whole Grains High in Polyphenols

1. Whole grain hard wheat flour

2. Whole grain rye flour

3. Whole grain wheat flour

4. Whole grain oat flour

Cacao Products High in Polyphenols

1. Cocoa powder

2. Dark chocolate

3. Milk chocolate

Wines High in Polyphenols

1. Red wine

2. White wine

3. Rosé wine

BEYOND NUTRITION

EXERCISE

About half of the studies looking at physical activity show that it keeps telomeres healthy, but the other half found no association. Given the many well-established benefits of exercise and the very real potential for telomere benefit, there are plenty of reasons to recommend moving more. For one, a habit of moderate exercise helps lower oxidative stress levels by inducing an antioxidant response to the temporary increases in oxidation caused by exercise. Think of it as good stress.

Some studies showed that runners had longer telomeres. Other studies demonstrated that people who got the most exercise each week had the healthiest telomeres. Still other studies found a protective effect with moderate activity. Interestingly, young athletes who trained intensively had longer telomeres than their peers, but middle-aged endurance runners showed signs of accelerated aging the more years and hours of training they had. Another study found that high-intensity cycling boosted telomeres more than moderate cycling for the same length of time. We don't know enough yet to recommend an exact amount or type of exercise for optimal telomere health, but it stands to reason to seek out a variety of enjoyable activity that includes cardio and strength training.

There's some evidence that exercise can increase telomerase activity, which helps telomeres self-heal and elongate. This was seen in a small group of healthy young males who ran at 80% of their maximum ability. Telomerase increased immediately afterward, and molecules that keep telomeres healthy were elevated for an hour after exercise. This was replicated in other small studies that included men and women. However, as seen in a 6-month study of caregivers, the immediate effect didn't last. Still, there seemed to be long-term benefits. This study found that those who did aerobic activity for 40 minutes three to five times a week had longer telomeres than their sedentary peers.

The highest level of recommended activity described in the Physical Activity Guidelines for Americans is 1,000 MET-minutes per week, although the guidelines note that greater levels of activity yield greater benefits. MET stands for metabolic equivalent, a unit of energy expenditure: 1 MET is the rate of energy expended at rest, and a 2-MET activity uses twice the energy as the body uses at rest. MET-minutes are used to measure activity in research because they make it easy to standardize and compare different activities. This method considers the level of activity as well as the duration. For example, a 30-minute walk and a 15-minute run could reasonably equal the same MET-minutes. To get to total MET-minutes, multiply the level of MET by the length of an activity. For example, a 3-MET activity done for 30 minutes equals 90 MET-minutes; a 2-MET activity done for 45 minutes also equals 90 MET-minutes.

Text continued on page 96.

Physical Activity Measured in METs

ACTIVITY	METs	EXAMPLE	MINUTES NEEDED to get to 1,375 MET-minutes per week (women)
Bicycling	8	Bicycling, general	171.9
Conditioning	2.5	Mild stretching	550.0
Conditioning	7	Stationary bike, general	196.4
Conditioning	3	Stationary bike, 50 watts, very light effort	458.3
Conditioning	5.5	Stationary bike, 100 watts, light effort	250.0
Conditioning	7	Stationary bike, 150 watts, moderate effort	196.4
Conditioning	10.5	Stationary bike, 200 watts, vigorous effort	131.0
Conditioning	12.5	Stationary bike, 250 watts, very vigorous effort	110.0
Conditioning	3.5	Calisthenics home exercise, light to moderate effort	392.9
Conditioning	8	Calisthenics (push-ups, sit-ups, pull-ups, jumping jacks), heavy, vigorous effort	171.9
Conditioning	8	Circuit training, minimal rest	171.9
Conditioning	6	Weight lifting	229.2
Conditioning	9	Stair-treadmill	152.8
Dancing	8.5	Step aerobics with a 6–8" step	161.8
Dancing	10	Step aerobics with a 10–12" step	137.5
Dancing	4.5	Disco, folk, square, line, polka, contra, country	305.6
Dancing	4.8	Ballet, modern, twist, jazz, tap, jitterbug	286.5
Dancing	5.5	Ballroom, fast	250.0

HOURS PER WEEK	MINUTES PER DAY	MINUTES NEEDED to get to 1,887 MET-minutes per week (men)	HOURS PER WEEK	MINUTES PER DAY
2.9	25	236	3.9	34
9.2	79	755	12.6	108
3.3	28	270	4.5	39
7.6	65	629	10.5	90
4.2	36	343	5.7	49
3.3	28	270	4.5	39
2.2	19	180	3.0	26
1.8	16	151	2.5	22
6.5	56	539	9.0	77
2.9	25	236	3.9	34
2.9	25	236	3.9	34
3.8	33	315	5.2	45
2.5	22	210	3.5	30
2.7	23	222	3.7	32
2.3	20	189	3.1	27
5.1	44	419	7.0	60
4.8	41	393	6.6	56
4.2	36	343	5.7	49

Physical Activity Measured in METs

ACTIVITY	METs	EXAMPLE	MINUTES NEEDED to get to 1,375 MET-minutes per week (women)
Dancing	3	Ballroom, slow (waltz, foxtrot, samba, tango, mambo, cha-cha)	458.3
Fishing and hunting	3	Fishing	458.3
Home	3.5	Mopping	392.9
Home	2.5	Multiple activities done in one bout, light effort	550.0
Home	3.5	Multiple activities done in one bout, moderate effort	392.9
Home	4	Multiple activities done in one bout, vigorous effort	343.8
Home	3.5	Vacuuming	392.9
Home	2.5	Watering plants	550.0
Home	3	Carrying small children	458.3
Home	4	Elder care, disabled adults, only active periods	343.8
Inactivity	1	Lying quietly, lying in bed awake, listening to music (not talking or reading), sitting quietly, watching a movie	1,375.0
Lawn and garden	4	Raking lawn	343.8
Lawn and garden	3	Picking fruits and vegetables, moderate effort	458.3
Miscellaneous	2	Standing	687.5
Miscellaneous	1.5	Sitting, arts and crafts, light effort	916.7
Miscellaneous	2	Sitting, arts and crafts, moderate effort	687.5

HOURS PER WEEK	MINUTES PER DAY	MINUTES NEEDED to get to 1,887 MET-minutes per week (men)	HOURS PER WEEK	MINUTES PER DAY
7.6	65	629	10.5	90
7.6	65	629	10.5	90
6.5	56	539	9.0	77
9.2	79	755	12.6	108
6.5	56	539	9.0	77
5.7	49	472	7.9	67
6.5	56	539	9.0	77
9.2	79	755	12.6	108
7.6	65	629	10.5	90
5.7	49	472	7.9	67
22.9	196	1,887	31.5	270
5.7	49	472	7.9	67
7.6	65	629	10.5	90
11.5	98	944	15.7	135
15.3	131	1,258	21.0	180
11.5	98	944	15.7	135

Physical Activity Measured in METs

ACTIVITY	METs	EXAMPLE	MINUTES NEEDED to get to 1,375 MET-minutes per week (women)
Miscellaneous	1.8	Standing, arts and crafts, light effort	763.9
Miscellaneous	3	Standing, arts and crafts, moderate effort	458.3
Miscellaneous	3.5	Standing, arts and crafts, vigorous effort	392.9
Running	4.5	Jogging on mini-trampoline	305.6
Walking	3	Walking the dog	458.3
Walking	8	Walking briskly, 5 mph	171.9

NHANES data show that significantly longer telomeres in women and men were not apparent until women reached at least 1,375 MET-minutes per week, and men at least 1,887 MET-minutes per week. At these MET-minute levels, women and men were nine years biologically younger than their sedentary peers who were otherwise similar in age, gender, race, education, BMI, smoking status, and level of alcohol use. These findings were based on nearly 6,000 U.S. adults, ages 20 to 84 years and representative of the population.

In order for a woman to reach 1,375 MET-minutes per week, she could ride her bike for 25 minutes a day, do 20 minutes of step aerobics with a 10- to 12-inch step, walk the dog for a little more than an hour a day, or some combination of these activities and others. For a man to reach 1,887 MET-minutes per week, he could do 22 minutes a day of vigorous riding on a stationary bike, a little more than half an hour a day of brisk walking at 5 miles per hour, or an hour of country or folk dancing. Check out the table starting on page 92 for more examples of METs for

HOURS PER WEEK	MINUTES PER DAY	MINUTES NEEDED to get to 1,887 MET-minutes per week (men)	HOURS PER WEEK	MINUTES PER DAY
12.7	109	1,048	17.5	150
7.6	65	629	10.5	90
6.5	56	539	9.0	77
5.1	44	419	7.0	60
7.6	65	629	10.5	90
2.9	25	236	3.9	34

common activities and the equivalent time needed to reach the level found in the research.

A combination of physical activity and meditation such as yoga may offer unique benefits beyond exercise alone. A 2017 study of 96 healthy adults found that 12 weeks of yoga improved telomerase activity along with other markers of aging. Although there was a trend toward increased telomere length, the findings were not statically significant. It may mean there was no effect, or it could mean that the number of people in the study was too small or the length of time too short to find meaningful results. Regardless, the improved telomerase activity is promising, especially as it was accompanied by significantly lower markers of DNA damage, the main stress hormone cortisol, and inflammatory markers along with higher levels of cellular aging protectors such as antioxidant capacity and neuron-protecting brain-derived neurotrophic factor (BDNF).

STRESS MANAGEMENT

In a 2018 randomized clinical trial of 53 adults ages 50 to 84 years with subjective cognitive decline, researchers found that a 12-week relaxation program improved telomere length and telomerase activity, cognitive function, sleep, mood, and quality of life. Each participant had experienced a cognitive deficit within the previous six months, could give an example of memory lapses that interrupted their everyday life, and had these lapses at least once a week, but didn't have overt cognitive deficits such as the inability to follow simple directions or complete questionnaires. Still, the participants felt they had declined in the past 5 to 10 years and were worried about it (ironically, something that increases the risk of cognitive decline).

Telomere, telomerase, cognitive, and psychosocial measures were taken at baseline, after the three-month program, and then at six months (three months after the program period concluded). The relaxation program consisted of 12 minutes a day of either meditation or listening to music. Participants in both the meditation and music groups improved memory and cognitive function at three and six months. They also had greater telomerase activity if they followed at least two-thirds of the program, the equivalent of four days a week or about every other day. The meditation group saw better improvements in stress, mood, and quality of life mental health than the group that listened to music. People with shorter telomeres saw bigger improvements in telomere length. The increases in telomere length and telomere activity were associated with improvements in mood, stress, health-related quality of life, memory, and cognitive performance.

Meditation and Music Therapy

Both programs asked participants to sit comfortably with their eyes closed for 12 minutes a day for 12 weeks. The kind of meditation used for this intervention is a beginner's technique called Kirtan Kriya. It's as easy as 1-2-3: one, chant; two, touch; and three, visualize. All you have to do is repeat the chant, "Sa-Ta-Na-Ma" while touching the thumb to each fingertip with each chant, and visualizing energy coming into the body from the head and exiting between the eyebrows in an *L* shape.

The music therapy involved listening to relaxing instrumental music by six classical composers—Bach, Beethoven, Debussy, Mozart, Pachelbel, and Vivaldi. The music of each composer was played at least once during the 12 weeks.

The moral of this story is to spend less time worrying about cognitive decline, which is counterproductive, and more time focusing on relaxation. Daily is great, but every other day still has benefits, and all it takes is 12 minutes a day.

Resilience

As the old song made famous by Ella Fitzgerald goes, "Into each life, some rain must fall." Life isn't a stress-free experience, and banishing stress isn't even the goal. While we know that stress can negatively impact telomere health, *stress* is another word for *challenge*, and challenges can help us grow and improve. So what are we supposed to do about stress?

Well, some of that decision has been made for us because there are things in life we can't control. However, we are in control of how we react. Researchers have studied the link between resiliency to stress and telomere health. As described in a 2019 paper, caregivers with parenting stress (caring for a child with autism) who were able to integrate their challenges into a narrative identity for themselves, were able to improve markers for stress and telomere health.

WHAT IS NARRATIVE IDENTITY?

Narrative identity is an individual's sense of their own life story. It's when a person integrates a perception of their past and imagined future into a cohesive story line that provides unity and purpose to their life. Studies have found that people who find redemption and growth through past suffering and adversity to construct stories of their life themed around taking initiative and demonstrating curiosity tend to be more mature and enjoy better mental health and overall well-being. These are stories of optimism and finding the good in the bad. The well-being of people with more redemption stories in their life narrative tend to be greater.

Interestingly, the researchers found that coherent narratives were associated with improved telomere health and lower parenting stress over a year and a half, despite the kinds of themes that emerged. This suggests that learning to integrate the meaning of stressful experiences into a unified life view on its own is a way to improve the telomere health and stress of people under chronic stress. Creating a narrative is a way of showing agency, or active control, over a situation, which takes the place of helplessness and hopelessness common with depression.

Narrative identity may be an individual's story, but the individual does not need to be the hero of every part of it. That is called narcissism, and raises the self up while putting everyone else down. It doesn't have to be this way. In fact, people who tend to think about the well-being of future generations, often create stories about other people who have helped them along the way.

Meditation with Movement

Examples of meditation with movement include yoga and tai chi. This kind of meditation incorporates deep breathing, which on its own can bring calm if you can't make it to a yoga class.

Pay attention to breath and take purposeful, slow, deep, even breaths. It also incorporates autogenic training, which means being aware of the warmth, weight, and relaxation in different parts of the body. Often the end of a yoga class will include progressive relaxation, although this can also be done on its own. It involves tensing and relaxing muscle groups. In a yoga class, it's led by verbal cues, but you could do it on your own.

Not many clinical trials in this area exist, and sample sizes tend to be small. Exploratory research into mind-body interventions to help with distress, depression and stress, poor sleep, pain, and fatigue in cancer survivors is also exploring impact on telomere length and telomerase activity, although findings have not yet been published. The dozen or so randomized trials available on yoga and meditation and telomeres point to a positive impact on cellular aging. It may work by increasing the production of certain enzymes that thwart the buildup of reactive oxidant species (ROS, aka DNA-damaging free radicals). It dampens the hypothalamic-pituitary-adrenal stress response, which reduces oxidative activity.

Other Relaxation Techniques

If yoga isn't for you, there are many other ways to manage stress. Do what works for you. Some outside-the-box options include biofeedback, which uses electronic devices to provide immediate feedback to teach you how to relax tense muscles; guided imagery, which helps displace stressful thoughts with something more pleasant, and can be led by a coach or done on your own; and self-hypnosis, which you do on your own, prompted by something you choose, and puts your brain in the same state as daydreaming, deep meditation, or light sleep, lost in your thoughts. It could involve staring into a fire or at a painting. Another method is to sit quietly, breathing slowly, and repeating a positive mantra, and then slowly bringing yourself back into the world; you're never out of control.

PSYCHOSOCIAL HEALTH

The psychological and social factors in life include social support, personal control, symbolic meanings and norms, and mental health, and there are complex interconnections between all these factors. Supportive interactions with others have many health benefits: they boost immune, endocrine, and cardiovascular functions, and reduce the load of chronic stress responses. We also know that the sense that one is loved, cared for, and listened to goes a long way. It indirectly improves mental health through stress reduction and fostering a sense of meaning in life.

CARING BEHAVIORS BENEFIT GIVER AND RECIPIENT

Meaningful interactions with others can benefit the giver as much as the recipient. Caring behaviors include offers to help and expressions of affection, both without expectation of anything in return. Relationships are often with our family members and life partners, but they can also be with organizations such as a religious institution or volunteer organization.

Social isolation can increase the risk for age-related disease, especially if people feel a loss or lack of meaningful relationships. In a bird study, social isolation was found to shorten telomeres. In human studies across nations, those with the lowest involvement in social relationships were more likely to die. In adults with coronary artery disease, those who were socially isolated were 2.4 times as likely to die than their more connected peers. It's not just about how often you connect with others, but also the quality of healthy habits you engage in together.

Many studies suggest that having a strong network of people who provide emotional support is associated with longer telomeres, although other study found the opposite or no association. Studies of social ties and cellular aging are in their infancy, and disparate findings come with different samples and measures.

May I suggest, be loving, let your love language be healthy habits for yourself and others, show others you care for them, and witness and listen to their life.

CHAPTER 4

THE FOUR-WEEK JUMP-START TELOMERE HEALTH PLAN

HOW TO USE THIS JUMP-START GUIDE

This is called a jump-start plan because it's a short four weeks. Each week focuses on one healthy action you can take to keep your telomeres healthy, with fringe benefits for your heart, brain, and general well-being. Resist the temptation to change everything at once. That's why the weeks have separate emphases. It's because I want you to succeed.

Making small changes, and attacking each change fervently, is the way to go. Small changes are amazing and lead to big results. Setting your sights on a goal or desired result without an actionable plan is ineffective. That's because there's a difference between results and actions, and the difference means everything. Results are dreams. Actions are real. Actions get you to your dreams. If you learn to enjoy the process, the results will come on their own.

I encourage you to focus on one change for as long as you need—or to go back to certain weeks whenever you need and stay there for a while. Don't let all the changes overwhelm you by tackling them all at once. As one new behavior becomes comfortable, you'll know you're ready to add more change.

This is your plan of action:

Start with the self-assessment.

Week 1: Focus on sleep rituals because changing something binary (you're either asleep or you're not) is the easiest tactic for moving forward on your path of wellness, although it does still require effort.

Week 2: Explore relaxation and self-reflective caring behaviors.

Week 3: Make time for exercise and physical activity.

Week 4: Be mindful of nourishment by following the sample meal plan.

It may seem strange to end with food in a book about nutrition, but the truth is that what and how we eat is a very complex set of habits to shift. Having the other elements in place will make it easier to succeed. And you will be great at this. But you still have to eat for the first three weeks, so if you want to peruse the recipes and try any of them along the way, feel free to do so. Just don't feel the need to change everything about what you're eating from the get-go.

WHAT YOU'VE LEARNED SO FAR

If you've read from the first page to here, you know a little something about telomeres and telomerase, how they don't mix well with inflammation and oxidative stress, and how what you eat and other lifestyle factors can impact your life for better or for worse. If you need a quick refresher, here are the highlights:

Telomeres are strands of noncoding DNA that sit on the ends of your chromosomes, protecting and stabilizing the chromosomal DNA, which is what makes you *you*.

Telomeres diminish every time cells divide until they become so short that they can't do a proper job of protecting the DNA in chromosomes.

Some telomere shortening is normal, and some is premature and avoidable.

Shorter telomeres are associated with aging, and very short telomeres are associated with disease and early death.

Telomerase is an enzyme that can form, maintain, and restore length to telomeres, which can be positive (slowing down biological aging on a cellular level) or negative (cancer).

Most of your telomere length is inherited, but not all, and your lifestyle can do a lot to impact the part that's not inherited.

Inflammation and oxidative stress are known to shorten and erode telomeres prematurely. The things that elevate inflammation and oxidative stress, such as unhealthy foods, poor sleep habits, lack of exercise, negative reactions to stress, and exposure to smoke and pollution, all contribute to prematurely unraveling your telomeres and accelerating how quickly you age.

I repeat, lifestyle can play a big role in impacting the health of your telomeres.

Although telomere science is relatively new, never forget that all the healthy habits in this jump-start guide are backed by established, sound science for heart health, diabetes prevention, digestive health, cognitive function, and all-around well-being.

SELF-ASSESSMENT

Research suggests that many factors can influence the health of telomeres, and therefore an assessment of lifestyle habits that may be helping or hurting your telomeres should integrate multiple factors, from your eating habits to your interpersonal relationships. This self-assessment is not a clinical tool but is designed as a simple, quick way to help you recognize areas that could use improvement. Work toward a score of 14 to 28.

Self-Assessment

	NEVER (0 points)	SOMETIMES (1 point)	ALWAYS (2 points)
5–9 servings of fruits and vegetables (includes 100% juice) every day			
Whole grains every day			
Fish or seaweed (not fried) twice a week			
Coffee or tea every day			
Olive oil your main fat			

	NEVER (0 points)	SOMETIMES (1 point)	ALWAYS (2 points)
Nuts every day			
Beans every other day			
30–60 minutes of exercise every day			
No smoking			
No more than 1 alcoholic drink per day for women, 2 for men			
Sleep 7 hours or more every day			
Regular sleep ritual			
Regular stress management activities			
Regular caring behaviors toward others and self			
TOTAL (28 points possible)			

WEEK 1: YOUR SLEEP RITUAL

Sleep gives your brain time to flush away metabolic waste, your breathing relaxes, your heart rate lowers to give your heart a break, and your muscles release growth hormones for rebuilding and repairing.

First and foremost, work with a qualified health professional to resolve any medical issues getting in the way of a good night's sleep, such as obstructive sleep apnea. Then develop your own sleep guidelines and ritual. Try different strategies and see what works best for you.

These tips are adapted from the National Sleep Foundation:

1. Set a bedtime as well as a wake time. Be consistent, even on weekends. Write down your bed time and wake time below.

Bedtime: _____

Wake time: _____

2. Starting four to six hours before bedtime, avoid eating or drinking anything that may keep you awake. This includes stimulants such as caffeine (e.g., regular coffee or tea, chocolate, caffeinated sodas) and nicotine (and consider a cessation program). Alcohol, which can make you feel drowsy, leads to poor-quality sleep and often waking up less rested. Drinking too many liquids may lead to bathroom trips in the evening. Heavy greasy foods can lead to reflux if you lie down too quickly after eating, and that leads to discomfort and poor sleep.

Going to bed too hungry can also keep you up later, so plan on a light snack one to two hours before bedtime. Some ideas: apples and peanut butter, a glass of milk, a small cup of oatmeal and fruit. Below, write down some ideas for a healthy snack, and the time you'll eat it.

Pre-bedtime snack: _____

Time: _____

3. Create a peaceful bedroom that is quiet, cool, and dark. No screens. If noise bothers you, use earplugs. Try a white noise machine (or app) if too much quiet keeps you up. If light gets in, try room-darkening shades. Keep your sheets and pillow cases clean, washing them at least weekly. Replace your pillows every year or two, and your mattress every 10 years or so. If you enjoy aromatherapy, use calming essential oils such as sage, lavender, or marjoram on your forehead or pulse points before bed. Write down at least one idea you will try this week.

Peaceful bedroom ideas:

4. Develop a winding-down ritual to help you relax each night. It can be a warm shower, reading, or listening to calming music. Avoid screens, which are stimulating. No TV. Instead, consider a meditation activity. There are apps with soothing, sometimes purposefully monotone and soothing words read out loud to help you drift off. Try slow breathing. Write down the ideas you'd like to try this week.

Winding-down ritual ideas:

5. Don't fixate on the fact that you're awake. Don't stare at the clock. Instead, turn to a relaxation technique from your winding-down ritual. Write down some ideas so you have a plan if this happens to you.

Fall-back technique if you can't sleep:

Write down the steps you'll take to practice healthy sleep habits this week. You'll probably want to start by creating a peaceful environment in your bedroom, so I filled in that one for you.

Week 1: Your Sleep Ritual

DAY 1	Create a peaceful bedroom.
DAY 2	
DAY 3	
DAY 4	
DAY 5	
DAY 6	
DAY 7	

WEEK 2: RELAXATION AND SELF-CARE

Relaxation strategies to relieve stress tend to be generally safe and low-cost for most people, which makes them a low-risk therapy to embark upon. The potential for upside is excellent, from relieving anxiety and insomnia to managing headaches, nausea, and chronic pain. Ultimately, the goal is to slow breathing, lower blood pressure, and improve mood and well-being.

	WEEK 2: RELAXATION AND SELF-CARE	YOUR PLAN
DAY 1	15 minutes of listening to calming music with eyes closed	
DAY 2	Practice "invisible" caring. Do something to help someone else, with no expectation of thanks.	
DAY 3	12 minutes of chant-touch-visualize exercise, Kirtan Kriya (page 98)	
DAY 4	15 minutes of listening to calming music with eyes closed	
DAY 5	5 minutes of deep breathing	
DAY 6	Think of something in your life that has brought you stress. Write it down. Think about who helped you overcome it. Write about it. Read more about creating your narrative identity below.	

WEEK 2: RELAXATION AND SELF-CARE	YOUR PLAN
DAY 7 Share the story you developed yesterday with someone. Ask them how they are and listen to their story. Read more about sharing your story below.	

CREATING YOUR NARRATIVE IDENTITY

This is not just a collection of facts and events that have happened in your life. Rather, it weaves all these points together to create meaning. It doesn't just say what happened, but it says why, and it can reflect and shape who you are. A classic American story is to "study hard, go to college, get a good job, find your life partner, have a family"—but plenty of other paths are equally valid.

In stories about stress and challenges, how does the story unfold in your mind. What were common themes and what was your role in this story? Redemption stories are about something that starts poorly and ends well (every romantic comedy or, say, a horrible family vacation that ends up bringing everyone together). Contamination stories are about something that starts great and ends poorly (every horror movie). Do you have a contamination story in your life that you can reverse the script on? See how you can find the good and turn it into a redemption story.

Contamination story:

_____

_____

_____

_____

Redemption version:

_____

_____

_____

_____

Think of a story where you experienced redemption through your own strength and skills:

Now think of one where someone helped you through a hard time:

_____

_____

_____

_____

SHARE YOUR STORY

Tell someone your story because this will give you story muscle memory that will solidify and become part of your identity. Don't be afraid to tell your story and change it according to feedback. Outside input can give you new things to think about as well as add a level of flexibility to your own story and opportunity for growth.

WEEK 3: EXERCISE AND PHYSICAL ACTIVITY

Women: Aim for 1,375 MET-minutes per week

Men: Aim for 1,887 MET-minutes per week

Review the MET values for various activities on page 92, and make your own plan for Week 3 or use the one below.

Week 3: Exercise and Physical Activity

	ACTIVITY	YOUR PLAN	MET-MINUTES
DAY 1	Bike ride, 25 minutes		
DAY 2	Brisk walk, 40 minutes		
DAY 3	Yoga, 60 minutes		
DAY 4	Step aerobics, 20 minutes		
DAY 5	Brisk walk, 40 minutes		
DAY 6	Dancing, 60 minutes		
DAY 7	Housecleaning, 60 minutes		
TOTAL WEEKLY MET-MINUTES:			

WEEK 4: NOURISHMENT

This week's focus is on eating mindfully. Say yes to fruits, vegetables, nuts, seafood, legumes, whole grains, and other healthy foods.

While the snack is listed after dinner in the sample meal plan, you can have a snack anytime throughout the day.

Week 4: Sample Meal Plan

DAY 1
Breakfast: Rainbow Carrot Shakshuka (page 122)

Lunch: Roasted Carrot Sandwich (page 148) with Couscous with Grapes and Snow Peas (page 162)

Dinner: Pistachio-Crusted Chicken (page 169) with Lemony Asparagus (page 157). Put a portion of dinner away for tomorrow's lunch.

Anytime Snack: Gimbap (page 154)

Notes: Buy enough carrots to make today's breakfast and lunch.

DAY 2
Breakfast: Avocado Toast (page 121)

Lunch: Leftover chicken and asparagus

Dinner: Chickpea-Stuffed Sweet Potatoes (page 182). Put a portion of dinner away for tomorrow's lunch.

Anytime Snack: Leftover gimbap

Notes: Buy sweet potatoes once, and make two dinners today and tomorrow.

DAY 3

Breakfast: Avocado Toast

Lunch: Leftover chickpea dish

Dinner: Turkey Sweet Potato Stew (page 137). Put a portion of dinner away for tomorrow's lunch; label, date, and freeze any extras.

Anytime Snack: Sweet and Spicy Mango Cheeks (page 150)

DAY 4

Breakfast: Get Your Greens Smoothie (page 127)

Lunch: Leftover stew

Dinner: Harissa-Spiced Striped Bass (page 178) with Garlicky Summer Squash (page 159). Put a portion of dinner away for tomorrow's lunch.

Anytime Snack: Pears with Yogurt Dip (page 152)

Notes: Prep the overnight oats for tomorrow's breakfast.

DAY 5

Breakfast: Mason Jar Overnight Oats (page 126)

Lunch: Leftover striped bass and squash

Dinner: Taco Bowl (page 170). Put a portion of dinner away for tomorrow's lunch.

Anytime Snack: Balsamic-Fig Nice Cream (page 192)

DAY 6

Breakfast: 5-Minute Egg Toast (page 124)

Lunch: Leftover taco bowl

Dinner: Sheet Pan Salmon (page 174). Put a portion of dinner away for tomorrow's lunch.

Anytime Snack: Matcha-Ginger Chia Pudding (page 191)

DAY 7

Breakfast: Breakfast Tacos (page 125)

Lunch: Leftover salmon

Dinner: Butternut Squash and Ginger Soup (page 134) with Couscous with Grapes and Snow Peas (page 162)

Anytime Snack: Quickle Rainbow Carrots (page 156)

Notes: Label, date, and freeze any extra soup.

WEEKLY SHOPPING LIST

Your shopping list will change from week to week depending on what you decide to make, but this is a solid starter list that will keep you stocked with healthy choices. These foods are on my own weekly shopping list and listed according to highest to lowest frequency of use.

Produce

❑ Apples, mandarin oranges, pears, nectarines for snacking

❑ Carrots, celery, cucumbers for snacking and salads

❑ Bananas for smoothies and banana bread

❑ Leafy greens such as kale, chard, romaine

❑ Onions, garlic

Meat and Seafood
- ❑ Salmon, halibut, tuna

- ❑ Skinless chicken breasts

- ❑ Lean ground turkey

Frozen
- ❑ Mixed dark berries

- ❑ Peas, broccoli, spinach

Staples
- ❑ Extra-virgin olive oil

- ❑ Green tea

- ❑ Almond milk

- ❑ Pistachios, almonds, walnuts

- ❑ Quinoa, farro, brown or wild rice

- ❑ Canned goods: tomatoes, tomato paste, beans

- ❑ Turmeric, chile powder

Supplements
Choose food first, but if you need a little help, consider supplements of vitamin B12, vitamin D, and omega-3 fatty acids (Nordic Naturals or Carlson). If using a multivitamin, choose one that is low in iron.

CHAPTER 5

RECIPES

Avocado Toast

Time: < 30 minutes   **Serves:** 2

2 slices whole wheat sourdough bread

1 small radish

2 teaspoons apple cider vinegar

1 small ripe avocado

sesame seeds, nori strips (optional)

lemon wedges

salt and pepper, to taste

1. Toast the bread.

2. Meanwhile, cut the radish in half lengthwise and thinly slice each piece into half moons.

3. In a small bowl, combine the radish slices and vinegar, tossing to coat. Set aside.

4. Cut the avocado lengthwise by slicing from the stem until you hit the seed, then rotate the knife carefully around the entire avocado. With your hands, rotate the two halves in opposite directions to pull them apart. Remove the seed by wedging a knife into it, rotating, and pulling (or scoop it out carefully with a thin spoon).

5. Use the "knick and peel" method to retain the most antioxidants from the dark green edge of the avocado flesh. Knick the stem off and peel the skin away. This works best with a ripe avocado. Repeat with the other avocado half.

6. Slice the avocado widthwise and divide evenly on the two slices of toast. Mash gently with a fork to spread. Top with the radish slices. Garnish with sesame seeds and nori strips, if using. Serve with a lemon wedge on the side or squeeze the juice over the toast to keep the avocado from browning. Season with salt and pepper to taste, and serve immediately.

Rainbow Carrot Shakshuka

Time: 30 to 60 minutes   **Serves:** 4 to 6

1 tablespoon extra-virgin olive oil, plus more as needed

1 small onion, diced

3 cups chopped rainbow carrots (5–8 medium carrots)

1 bunch chard, stems chopped and leaves thinly sliced into ribbons

2 medium tomatoes on the vine, diced

1 (15-ounce) can butter beans, drained and rinsed

¼ teaspoon ground turmeric

¼ teaspoon sumac

½ cup water

4 eggs

1 lemon

5 stems fresh flat-leaf parsley, leaves only, to garnish

salt and pepper, to taste

1. Heat 1 tablespoon oil in a large nonstick skillet over medium heat until hot but not smoking. Add the onion, and stir occasionally, until just wilted, about 2 minutes.

2. Stir in the carrots and chard stems, and season with salt and pepper. Cook, stirring occasionally, until the vegetables start to soften, about 5 minutes.

3. Add the tomatoes, beans, and chard leaves, and stir to combine.

4. Season with turmeric, sumac, and salt and pepper. Add the water, stir to combine, then cover to wilt the greens, about 2 to 3 minutes.

5. Uncover, make four indentations with the back of a spoon, and gently place an egg in each indentation. For best results, individually crack the eggs into separate bowls before pouring. Cook uncovered until the egg whites are just set, about 10 to 15 minutes.

6. Cut the lemon in half, remove seeds. Squeeze the juice from half the lemon over the cooked dish. Cut the other half into four wedges.

7. Garnish with parsley. If desired, finish with a drizzle of olive oil, and salt and pepper to taste. Serve warm with lemon wedges on the side.

Tip: If you can't find rainbow carrots, any kind of carrots work in this recipe.

5-Minute Egg Toast

Time: < 30 minutes   **Serves:** 1

1 slice whole grain bread

1 egg

1 tablespoon water (optional)

2 tablespoons hummus

2 tablespoons chopped red bell pepper

red chile flakes (optional)

salt and pepper, to taste

1. Toast the bread.

2. Meanwhile, in a medium microwave-safe bowl, whisk the egg (add the water for a fluffier egg), and season with salt and pepper.

3. Microwave the egg for 1 minute.

4. Spread the hummus on toast, sprinkle with the bell pepper, and top with the egg. Season with chile flakes, if using, and salt and pepper to taste.

Breakfast Tacos

Time: 30 to 60 minutes   **Serves:** 4

4 eggs

2 small limes

1 medium tomato, medium dice

1 small avocado, medium dice

¼ bunch fresh cilantro (about ½ cup, loosely packed), chopped, divided

1 clove garlic, minced

1 tablespoon olive oil, plus more as needed

½ cup fresh, canned, or cooked from frozen sweet corn

½ cup black beans, drained and rinsed

4 small corn tortillas

salt and pepper, to taste

1. Bring a medium pot of water to a boil over high heat. Add the eggs and boil for 5 to 7 minutes to soft-boiled doneness. While the eggs are cooking, prepare an ice bath. Plunge the cooked eggs into the ice bath and let cool.

2. Meanwhile, zest the limes, juicing one and cutting the other into quarters. Pour the juice into a large bowl, and add the tomato, avocado, half the lime zest, half the cilantro, garlic, and 1 tablespoon oil. Fold in the corn and beans. Season with salt and pepper to taste.

3. Warm the tortillas, 1 to 2 minutes per side, in a nonstick skillet over medium heat. Set aside in a bowl covered with a paper towel or clean cloth towel.

4. When the eggs are cool enough to handle, peel and slice in half lengthwise.

5. Bring the tortillas, vegetable mixture, eggs, the other half of the cilantro, and the lime wedges to the table and assemble the tacos to your preference. As an alternative, place the tortillas on individual plates, add a couple of spoonfuls of the vegetable mixture to each tortilla, top with two egg halves, garnish with cilantro, and place a lime wedge on the side.

Mason Jar Overnight Oats

Time: < 30 minutes **Serves:** 1

⅓ cup old-fashioned rolled oats

⅓ cup blueberries

2 teaspoons chia seeds

¾ cup unsweetened vanilla almond-coconut milk

1 teaspoon roughly chopped pistachios

1 teaspoon cacao nibs

pinch of cinnamon

1. In a 2-cup mason jar with measurement markings, combine the oats, blueberries, and chia seeds. Top with enough almond-coconut milk (about ¾ cup) to reach the 1-cup mark on the jar. Stir gently. Cover and chill in refrigerator for at least 30 minutes, or overnight.

2. When ready to eat, top with the pistachios, cacao nibs, and cinnamon.

Get Your Greens Smoothie

Time: < 30 minutes   **Serves:** 2

2 frozen ripe bananas, broken into a few pieces

1 cup frozen mixed dark berries (blueberries, raspberries, blackberries)

2 leaves chard or kale, stems removed, leaves torn

1 cup milk or favorite unsweetened plant-based milk

½ teaspoon vanilla extract

1. Layer all the ingredients in a high-powered blender in the order listed.

2. Blend until smooth.

3. Pour into two glasses and serve immediately or refrigerate in an airtight container for up to 2 days.

Tip: *If you want to use smoothies as a leafy greens delivery vehicle, use this simple formula: 1 part leafy green + 1 part liquid + 1½ to 2 parts ripe fruit. For example, 1 cup baby spinach + 1 cup almond milk + 1 cup frozen mango + 1 frozen banana (about ½ cup).*

Tip: *To reduce food waste, save chard or kale stems; chop them up for another use. For example, heat a little olive oil in a small nonstick skillet until hot but not smoking. Add the stems and season with your favorite herbs and spices, sauté until they start to shine and barely soften, 1 to 2 minutes. Whisk an egg and pour it over the stems. Either stir a little for a scramble or leave alone for an omelet. Cook until eggs are set, about 1 minute. Slide the finished mixture on top of a piece of toast and you have another healthy breakfast or snack.*

Berry Zinger Smoothie Bowl

Time: < 30 minutes   **Serves:** 2

Smoothie:

2 frozen ripe bananas

2 cups frozen mixed dark berries (blueberries, raspberries, blackberries)

½ inch fresh ginger

1 cup milk or favorite unsweetened plant-based milk

½ teaspoon vanilla extract

Toppings:

small sliced banana, kiwi sliced into half moons, or ⅓ cup fresh blueberries

2–3 tablespoons lightly crushed pistachios or 2–3 tablespoons lightly crushed almonds

2 teaspoons chia seeds, 2 teaspoons hemp seeds, and/or 2 teaspoons cacao nibs

1. Place all the smoothie ingredients in a high-powered blender or food processor and combine until smooth but not overly liquefied, about 1 minute. Divide into two bowls.

2. Divide your choice of toppings between the two bowls. If desired, include seasonal fruit or other nuts and seeds.

Tip: *Don't hassle with a paring knife to peel fresh ginger. Simply use a spoon and apply some pressure to get the skin off. This is a much easier way to get into all the nooks and crannies.*

Lentil Soup

Time: 30 to 60 minutes   **Serves:** 6

3 tablespoons olive oil

1 medium onion, chopped

1 jalapeño pepper, minced

1 (6-ounce) can tomato paste

5 cloves garlic, minced

1 teaspoon ground cumin

1 teaspoon dried oregano

1 teaspoon ground turmeric

1 teaspoon chile powder

¾ cup split red lentils

1 (16-ounce) can diced tomatoes

7 cups chicken broth or stock

2 cups shredded cooked chicken

zest and juice from 2 limes

3 sprigs fresh cilantro

salt and pepper, to taste

1. In a large pot, heat the oil over medium heat until hot but not smoking. Sauté the onion and jalapeño pepper until softened, 1 to 2 minutes. Add the tomato paste, garlic, cumin, oregano, turmeric, and chile powder, stirring frequently until fragrant, about 1 minute.

2. Add the lentils, tomatoes, and chicken broth or stock. Stir to combine, cover, and bring to a boil, then reduce to a simmer and cook for an additional 15 minutes, or until the lentils are cooked through.

3. Remove from the heat. Add the chicken, lime juice, and half the lime zest. Stir to combine. Season with salt and pepper. Garnish with cilantro leaves and the remaining lime zest.

Tip: This recipe is great way to use up leftover chicken, or a grocery store rotisserie chicken.

White Fish Stew

Time: 30 to 60 minutes   **Serves:** 2

2 medium carrots

2 stalks broccolini

1 lemon

2 (6-ounce) Alaskan halibut fillets

2 tablespoons olive oil, divided

1 cup vegetable or fish broth

½ cup white wine

3 tablespoons capers, drained and rinsed

¼ cup almonds, roughly chopped

4–6 cherry tomatoes, halved

1 teaspoon red chile flakes

2 tablespoons Magic Spicy Green Sauce (page 204)

salt and pepper, to taste

1. Scrub well or peel the carrots. Cut on the diagonal into 2-inch pieces. Chop the leafy floret ends of the broccolini into 2-inch pieces, and cut each stem into 1-inch pieces. Set aside.

2. Zest the lemon, then cut in half. Juice half of the lemon, and cut the other half into wedges. Set aside.

3. Pat dry the fish with paper towels. Cut into 1-inch cubes, then season with salt and pepper.

4. In a large nonstick pan, heat 1 tablespoon oil over medium heat until hot but not smoking. Add the carrots and the broccolini stems, season with salt and pepper, and cook until tender crisp, about 2 minutes. Add the lemon juice, broth, and white wine, and bring to a boil. Add the fish and broccolini florets, reduce to a simmer, and cook for 3 to 4 minutes. Turn the fish and cook for another 3 to 4 minutes or until opaque, cooked through, and easy to flake. Remove from the heat and season with salt and pepper.

5. Combine the capers, almonds, tomatoes, lemon zest, and 1 tablespoon oil. Season with as much of the chile flakes as you like, salt and pepper to taste.

6. Divide the stew between two bowls. Garnish with the caper mixture, and drizzle Magic Green Sauce over top.

Seaweed Soup

Time: 30 to 60 minutes   **Serves:** 2 to 4

1 ounce dried seaweed

1 tablespoon toasted sesame oil, plus more as needed

2 cloves garlic, minced

2 tablespoons soup soy sauce

2 cups fish, chicken, or vegetable broth or stock

1 cup water

cooked chicken or fish (optional)

sliced scallions, sesame seeds (optional)

salt and pepper, to taste

1. In a large bowl, cover the seaweed with cold water and soak for 10 minutes. It will make about 2 cups after hydrating. Drain, squeeze to remove excess water, and cut into 2-inch pieces.

2. In a large pot over medium heat, heat the oil until hot but not smoking, and sauté the seaweed for 2 minutes.

3. Add the garlic and soy sauce, and stir for another 2 minutes. Then pour in the broth or stock and water, and bring to a boil.

4. If using cooked fish or chicken, add it now. Shred the chicken or flake the fish before adding it. Reduce heat and simmer for 20 minutes.

5. Before serving, drizzle on sesame oil if desired, and add scallions and sesame seeds, if using.

Tip: You can find dried seaweed at Asian markets or online retailers; it is different from the snacking seaweed or seaweed used for making rice rolls. It is also called sea mustard, miyeok, or wakame. Toasted sesame oil is much darker and aromatic than regular sesame oil, and a little goes a long way, which is important to remember if you decide to drizzle a little on top before serving. Soup soy sauce is a type of

Korean soy sauce also known as guk-ganjang that is lighter in color so it won't overwhelm the color of a light soup. It is also saltier than regular soy sauce, so less is needed. This soup is a great way to use up a small amount of chicken or fish from a previous meal.

Butternut Squash and Ginger Soup

Time: 1 to 2 hours   **Serves:** 8

1 large (4-pound) butternut squash, cubed (yields 6–8 cups), seeds saved

1 tablespoon plus 1 teaspoon grapeseed oil, divided

1 tablespoon extra-virgin olive oil, or more as needed

1 medium yellow onion, roughly chopped

6 cloves garlic, roughly chopped

3 tablespoons curry powder

1 teaspoon chile flakes

½ cup raw cashews

8 ounces silken tofu

2 cups vegetable broth or stock

2 tablespoons chopped fresh ginger root

4 dried apricots, roughly chopped

½ recipe, Cashew Crema (page 213)

4 sprigs fresh cilantro, pulled into 8–16 pieces

salt and pepper, to taste

1. Preheat the oven to 400°F.

2. In a large bowl, toss the squash cubes with 1 tablespoon grapeseed oil. Season with salt and pepper to taste. Spread evenly on a sheet pan lined with foil, and roast for 20 minutes or until fork tender. Remove from the oven, and lower the heat to 275°F.

3. Heat 1 tablespoon olive oil in a large pot over medium heat. Sauté the onion until just fragrant, about 2 minutes. Add garlic and stir frequently until fragrant, about 30 seconds.

4. Add the curry powder and as much of the chile flakes as you like, season with salt and pepper to taste, and stir frequently until fragrant. Add more olive oil if the pan seems dry.

5. Add the squash, cashews, tofu, broth or stock, ginger, and apricots, and bring to a boil. Lower the heat and simmer for 15 minutes.

6. Meanwhile, spread the rinsed and dried squash seeds on a foil-lined sheet pan, and roast at 275°F for 15 minutes or until the seeds start to pop. Heat 1 teaspoon grapeseed oil in a small pan, and transfer the seeds, stirring constantly until one pops, about 1 minute. Season with salt and pepper. Set aside on a paper towel–lined plate.

7. Transfer the soup to a high-powered blender, in batches as needed, and blend until creamy and smooth. Return the soup to the pot. Taste and adjust seasonings.

8. Serve with a drizzle of Cashew Crema, roasted squash seeds, and cilantro.

Tip: *To prep the squash, cut it in two large pieces, where the narrow neck meets the bulb. Peel with a Y-peeler down to the orange flesh, peeling away all white flesh and green veins. Cut into approximately equal cubes. Clean, rinse and dry the seeds on a clean towel or paper towel, set aside (a fine-mesh strainer helps separate the seeds from the stringy flesh). Plain Greek yogurt or Icelandic skyr can sub in for the Cashew Crema.*

Spring Gazpacho

Time: 30 to 60 minutes   **Serves:** 4

2 pounds ripe tomatoes, roughly chopped

1 red bell pepper, roughly chopped

½ small red onion, roughly chopped

1 clove garlic

1 large cucumber, half roughly chopped and half diced, divided

¼ cup extra-virgin olive oil, plus more as needed

2 tablespoons sherry vinegar

salt and pepper, to taste

1. Combine the tomatoes, bell pepper, onion, garlic, roughly chopped cucumber half, and ¼ cup oil in a high-powered blender, and blend until smooth or to desired consistency.

2. Taste, then add the sherry vinegar. Taste again, and add salt and pepper to taste. Refrigerate until ready to serve.

3. To serve, divide among four bowls, garnish with the diced cucumber and a drizzle of good olive oil.

Tip: *Time is this recipe's friend—it tastes even better the day after. This is a great way to transform ripe vegetables that are on their last legs into something beautiful and delicious. Make substitutions as you wish; for example, a shallot for the red onion, your favorite vinegar or citrus juice for the sherry vinegar, or a fennel bulb, avocado, corn, peas, or anything that's in season for the bell pepper. This gazpacho goes great with a piece of country bread.*

Turkey Sweet Potato Stew

Time: 30 to 60 minutes   **Serves:** 2

1 tablespoon grapeseed oil

10 ounces ground turkey

¼ cup minced shallot
(1–2 shallots)

2 tablespoons tomato paste

1 tablespoon chile spice blend
(store-bought or recipe below)

1 medium sweet potato, diced

1 cup diced fresh tomato

½ cup canned black beans,
drained and rinsed

2 cups water, broth, or stock

½ small avocado, diced

2 sprigs fresh cilantro,
leaves roughly chopped

½ lime, cut into
2 wedges (optional)

salt and pepper, to taste

Spice Blend:

1 tablespoon gochugaru
or red chile flakes

1 teaspoon ground cumin

1 teaspoon ground coriander

½ teaspoon sweet
smoked paprika

½ teaspoon garlic powder

1. In a large pot, heat the oil over medium heat until hot but not smoking. Brown the ground turkey, breaking it into pieces and seasoning with salt and pepper, 2 to 3 minutes.

2. Add the shallot and stir constantly until softened, 2 to 3 minutes.

3. Add the tomato paste and chile spice blend, stirring constantly until the mixture is coated and fragrant, about 1 minute.

4. Add the sweet potato, tomato, beans, and water, broth, or stock. Taste and adjust the seasoning if needed. Bring to a boil, then reduce the heat and simmer for 20 minutes or until the sweet potato is tender and the liquid has thickened.

5. Serve in bowls and top with avocado, cilantro, and a lime wedge on the side, if using.

Samyetang

Time: 1 to 2 hours **Serves:** 2

½ cup Korean sweet rice

2 (1–2 pounds each) Cornish hens

8 cloves garlic, peeled

1 inch fresh ginger, roughly chopped

8 dried Korean red dates

9 cups water or chicken broth or stock

2 ginseng roots

2 astralagus roots

2 scallions, thinly sliced

salt and pepper, to taste

1. In a medium bowl, cover the rice with water and soak for an hour, then drain.

2. Meanwhile, pat dry the chicken with paper towels and season generously inside and out with salt. Let sit at room temperature for 30 to 60 minutes.

3. Combine the rice, garlic, ginger, and four of the dates. Stuff each hen with half the mixture.

4. In a large stock pot, cover the hens with the water or chicken broth or stock. Add the remaining four dates along with the ginseng and astralagus roots. Bring to a boil, then reduce to a simmer, cover and cook about an hour, or until the leg bones pull away easily but aren't falling apart.

5. In two large bowls, serve one hen, two dates, one ginseng root, and one astralagus root per person. Season with salt and pepper, and to taste. Garnish with scallions.

Tip: *Pick up an herb packet that includes astralagus from a Korean grocery store or online. Korean red dates, also known as jujubes, are redder and less sweet than the brown sticky sweet Medjool dates sold in most grocery stores. Note that Korean sweet rice is also called chapssal, or glutinous rice.*

Spring Greens and Soft-Boiled Eggs with Pistachios

Time: < 30 minutes   **Serves:** 4

4 eggs

2 cups sugar snap peas, trimmed, strings removed, and sliced on the diagonal

1 cup fresh or frozen peas

4 small radishes, quartered

1 baby fennel with fronds, bulb quartered and thinly sliced, ¼ cup fronds reserved

¼ cup French Vinaigrette (page 211)

1 cup pistachios

4 ounces goat cheese, crumbled

4 sprigs fresh mint, leaves only

¼ teaspoon paprika (optional)

1. In a medium pot, boil enough water to cover four eggs. Once at a rapid boil, reduce the heat to a simmer, add the eggs, bring the heat back up, and cook for 7 minutes. Meanwhile, prepare an ice bath. Transfer the cooked eggs to the ice bath to stop the cooking process. When cool enough to handle, peel and set aside.

2. In a large bowl, combine the snap peas, peas, radishes, and fennel slices, and toss with dressing.

3. In a food processor, pulse the pistachios to a coarse consistency. Set aside.

4. Divide the dressed salad evenly among four plates and top with the goat cheese and pistachio crumbs. Garnish with torn mint leaves and fennel fronds. To each plate, add one soft-boiled egg, cut in half lengthwise and sprinkled with paprika, if using.

Summer Salad

Time: 30 to 60 minutes   **Serves:** 4 to 6

1 cup uncooked farro

juice and zest from 1 lemon, divided, plus more as needed

3 tablespoons extra-virgin olive oil

1 head romaine lettuce

3 ripe plums, sliced

½ cup blueberries

3 medium tomatoes on the vine

4 sweet gypsy peppers, sliced into rings

1–2 ounces feta cheese

salt, pepper, and red chile flakes, to taste

1. Prepare the farro according to package directions for al dente result, drain, and set aside in a large bowl.

2. To make the dressing, whisk 2 tablespoons lemon juice with the oil, half the lemon zest, and salt, pepper, and red chile flakes, to taste. Set aside.

3. Tear the romaine leaves and add to the farro bowl. Toss with the dressing.

4. Fold in the plums, blueberries, tomatoes, sweet peppers, and the remaining lemon zest.

5. Garnish with the feta cheese and additional lemon zest, if using.

6. Season with salt and pepper just before serving.

Fall Fig and Fennel Raspberry-Kissed Salad

Time: < 30 minutes   **Serves:** 2 to 4

1 medium orange

4 cups lightly packed baby arugula

1 medium fennel bulb, bulb quartered and thinly sliced, fronds reserved

6 fresh figs, quartered lengthwise

Raspberry Vinaigrette (page 210)

salt and pepper, to taste

1. To prepare the orange, slice off the top and bottom, then with one flat side securely on the cutting board, slice away the remaining peel. Cut flesh-only segments. Squeeze the juice from what's left of the orange and whisk into the Raspberry Vinaigrette.

2. In a large serving dish, layer the arugula, fennel bulb slices, fennel fronds, orange segments, and figs. Drizzle with Raspberry Vinaigrette, and season with salt and pepper to taste. Serve immediately.

Tip: *Prewashed arugula works in this recipe. If you're not familiar with fennel, start by separating the bulb from the stalk. Then quarter the bulb. Cut out the tough root and heart with a diagonal slice and discard. Thinly slice the remaining white bulb on the diagonal to make thin strips.*

Winter Kale Salad

Time: 30 to 60 minutes   **Serves:** 8

2 cups uncooked farro

½ cup hazelnuts

1 bunch lacinato kale, leaves only, thinly sliced

Honey Dijon Vinaigrette (page 212)

3 tablespoons olive oil

1 medium yellow onion, finely diced

2 cups diced butternut squash

4 sprigs fresh thyme, leaves only, divided

2 tablespoons sherry vinegar

1 cup fresh pomegranate arils

salt and pepper, to taste

1. Preheat the oven to 350°F.

2. Prepare the farro according to package directions. Reserve 1 cup cooking liquid. Drain the farro and set aside.

3. Meanwhile, spread the hazelnuts in single layer on a baking sheet and toast in the oven for 5 to 7 minutes, until golden brown. Allow to cool slightly. Coarsely chop the nuts.

4. Massage the kale with a third of the Honey Dijon Vinaigrette for 3 to 5 minutes.

5. In a large pan over medium heat, heat the oil. Add the onion and cook until just tender, 2 to 3 minutes. Add the squash, season with salt and pepper, and cook, stirring occasionally, until tender, 8 to 10 minutes. Add the thyme, saving some for a garnish if desired, and cook for about 30 seconds. Remove from the heat. Stir in the vinegar. Transfer to a large mixing bowl. Fold in the farro, hazelnuts, and kale. Add some of the farro cooking liquid if the mixture seems dry. Gently fold in the pomegranate arils, saving some for a garnish if desired. Taste and adjust the seasoning if needed.

6. Transfer the mixture to a large serving bowl, garnish with any reserved thyme leaves and pomegranate arils, and serve, or cover and refrigerate for up to 2 days.

Tip: *You can substitute sweet potato or acorn squash for the butternut squash, and dried cranberries or fresh red grapes for the pomegranate arils. You can use leftover cooked squash; just heat it through for 2 to 3 minutes instead of cooking for 8 to 10.*

Watermelon Salad

Time: < 30 minutes   **Serves:** 4 to 6

1 small (3–5 pounds)
seedless watermelon,
about 8–10 cups diced

6 ounces sheep or
goat feta cheese

3–5 sprigs fresh mint,
torn, leaves only

zest and juice from 1 lemon

1 tablespoon extra-
virgin olive oil

salt and pepper, to taste

1. Place the diced watermelon in a large serving bowl.

2. Sprinkle the feta cheese and torn mint leaves on top. Add
the lemon zest and pour lemon juice over the salad.

3. Just before serving, season with salt and pepper and drizzle
the oil over top.

*Tip: Be sure to wash the outside of the watermelon before slicing,
which can spread anything on the outside of the fruit through the
flesh as you slice. To prepare the watermelon, cut in half widthwise.
Work on one half at a time. Set it on its flat cut-side down. Using a
downward motion, cut away the rind and pith until only the very red
flesh is showing.*

Pea Shoot, Egg, and Pickled Shallot Sandwich

Time: < 30 minutes   **Serves:** 2

2 eggs	¼ cup thinly sliced shallot
1–2 teaspoons red wine vinegar	2 slices whole grain sourdough bread
1 teaspoon olive oil	1 cup pea shoots
1 teaspoon honey	salt and pepper, to taste

1. Place the eggs in a small pot and cover with cold water. Heat over medium-low heat until boiling. Once boiling, turn the heat off, cover, and let sit for 12 minutes. With a slotted spoon, transfer to an ice bath. When cool enough to handle, peel and slice.

2. To pickle the shallot slices, whisk together the red wine vinegar, oil, honey, and salt and pepper in a small bowl. Add the shallot, tossing to combine. Stir every few minutes. Let marinate for at least 10 minutes, then drain before using.

3. Toast the bread. On top of each slice, evenly distribute the pea shoots, eggs slices, and pickled shallot. Serve as an open-faced sandwich, or fold in half and take it to go.

Tip: You can substitute baby arugula for the pea shoots, and red onion for the shallots.

Tofu Banh Mi

Time: 30 to 60 minutes **Serves:** 4

1 (14-ounce) package
extra-firm tofu, drained

2 cloves garlic

1 shallot

1 tablespoon fish sauce

½ teaspoon soy sauce,
plus more as needed

1 tablespoon plus 1 teaspoon
grapeseed oil, divided,
plus more as needed

1 inch fresh ginger or
lemongrass (optional)

3 medium Quickle Rainbow
Carrots (page 156)

4 tablespoons Greek yogurt

¼ teaspoon ground turmeric

1 whole grain baguette
(about 2 feet long)

1 small jalapeño pepper,
seeds removed, thinly sliced

1 cup thinly sliced on the
diagonal English cucumber

1 tablespoon chopped
fresh cilantro

1. Line a large baking sheet with paper towels and lay the tofu slices flat in one layer. Cover with additional paper towels and press gently until liquid soaks through. Replace the top paper towels and lay something heavy on top, such as another baking sheet, topped by heavy pots, plates, or even books. Wait at least 10 to 15 minutes before removing the paper towels. Once the tofu is compressed, slice into long ½-inch-thick slices.

2. To make the sauce, combine the garlic, shallot, fish sauce, ½ teaspoon soy sauce, 1 tablespoon oil, and ginger or lemongrass if using, in a food processor until coarsely chopped. Marinate the tofu in this sauce for at least 30 minutes and up to 2 hours.

3. Cut the Quickle Rainbow Carrots into 2- to 3-inch-long matchsticks.

4. Combine the yogurt and turmeric, and refrigerate until ready to use.

5. Cut the baguette into four sections, slice lengthwise nearly all the way through, and scoop out some of the inside of each section to make room for the filling. Toast the sections.

6. Meanwhile, cook the marinated tofu. Heat 1 teaspoon oil in a large nonstick pan over medium heat until hot but not smoking. Pat dry the tofu slices with paper towels before adding them to the pan, cooking 3 to 4 minutes per side until golden brown and warmed through, working in batches as needed. Add more oil if the pan seems dry between batches. Remove to a paper towel–lined plate.

7. Assemble the sandwich. Spread the yogurt-turmeric mixture on the bread, and add a few dashes of soy sauce. Building from the bottom up, layer the tofu, Quickle Rainbow Carrots, jalapeño pepper, cucumber, and cilantro. Serve any extra filling on the side.

Tip: *You can substitute tamari sauce or liquid aminos for the soy sauce, and vegetable or avocado oil for the grapeseed oil.*

Roasted Carrot Sandwich

Time: <30 minutes   **Serves:** 2

4 medium carrots

2 tablespoons olive oil

4 slices whole grain bread

4 tablespoons hummus
(store-bought or Red Beet
Hummus, page 206)

½ avocado, thinly sliced

¼ cup sprouts

1 lime, quartered

salt and pepper, to taste

1. Preheat the oven to 400°F.

2. Cut the carrots into logs about the same length as the short side of your bread, then slice in half lengthwise. Toss with the oil and salt and pepper. Spread on a sheet pan lined with foil and roast for 20 minutes.

3. Toast the bread.

4. Assemble the sandwiches. Spread 1 tablespoon hummus on each slice of bread. Divide the carrots between two slices, laying them flat side down on the bread. Divide the avocado between the other two slices of bread. Season with salt, pepper, and the juice from two lime wedges. Divide the sprouts and add on top of the avocado. Carefully place the slices with the carrots on top of the slices with the sprouts, and press gently. Slice the sandwiches on the diagonal, and serve with the remaining two lime wedges.

Pistachio-Crusted Rosemary and Fig Goat Cheese Boule

Time: 1 to 2 hours   **Serves:** 20

6 ounces soft goat cheese

4 ounces Neufchâtel cheese

7 ounces extra firm tofu, drained

½ cup dried figs, roughly chopped

2 sprigs fresh rosemary, leaves only, minced

¾ cup pistachio kernels, finely chopped

salt and pepper, to taste

1. In a large bowl, with gloved or clean hands, combine the goat cheese, Neufchâtel, and tofu until well blended.

2. Fold in the figs and rosemary, and evenly distribute them. Season with salt and pepper.

3. Shape into a ball (*boule* in French) and wrap in plastic wrap. Refrigerate for at least 1 hour.

4. Place the pistachios in a large bowl, and gently rotate the ball, pressing lightly to cover it with pistachios.

5. Place on a cheeseboard with a spreading knife and accompaniments such as almond crackers, sun-dried tomatoes, olives, fresh pears, and honeycomb.

Sweet and Spicy Mango Cheeks

Time: < 30 minutes   **Serves:** 1

1 medium mango	¼ teaspoon sumac
1 lime, cut into wedges	¼ teaspoon ground chile pepper

1. Place the mango on its long, thin side and carefully slice all the way through on either side of the seed to produce two "mango cheeks." Score each cheek to create ¾-inch squares. (If desired, cut the remaining flesh from the seed, and enjoy immediately or refrigerate for another use.)

2. Squeeze lime juice over the cheeks, and sprinkle with sumac and ground chile pepper.

Tip: *The easiest way to eat mango cheeks is with your hands. Simply invert the cheek so that the flesh pops out and take a bite. As an alternative, keep the fruit inverted and use a paring knife to cut away the fruit. Try eating the cheeks with pistachios or cashews, which are in the same botanical family as mango—and perhaps the reason they taste so good together.*

Pistachio Bites

Time: < 30 minutes   **Serves:** 5 to 8

25 red grapes

1 (5-ounce) container Greek yogurt or Icelandic skyr

½ cup crushed pistachios

25 toothpicks

1. Line a baking sheet with parchment paper.

2. Make sure the grapes are dry, then insert a toothpick into each one. Dip into the yogurt or skyr, then place on the parchment paper. Freeze for 15 minutes to soft-set.

3. Place the pistachios in a bowl. Remove the grapes from the freezer, and roll each in the pistachios to coat before returning it to the baking sheet.

4. Serve immediately or freeze in an airtight container for up to 2 months.

Tip: *Freeze the grapes for 2 to 3 hours before dipping to help the yogurt or skyr adhere better.*

Pears with Yogurt Dip

Time: < 30 minutes   **Serves:** 1

1 (5-ounce) container
Greek yogurt

1 tablespoon honey

¼ teaspoon cinnamon
(optional)

1 pear, any variety, sliced

1. In a bowl, stir the yogurt and honey together until well combined. Add the cinnamon, if using.

2. To enjoy, dip the pear slices in the yogurt dip.

Garnet Sweet Potato Toasts

Time: 30 to 60 minutes **Serves:** 4

1 medium garnet sweet potato

2 tablespoons plus ½ teaspoon olive oil, divided

¼ cup frozen raspberries

2 tablespoons balsamic vinegar

1 teaspoon honey

1 teaspoon chia seeds

4 tablespoons Greek yogurt

1 medium Fuyu persimmon, thinly sliced widthwise into rounds

4 teaspoons pomegranate arils

1 sprig fresh thyme, leaves only

salt and pepper, to taste

1. Preheat the oven to 400°F.

2. Slice the sweet potato lengthwise into four "toasts," each about ½ inch wide. You will end up with two thin lengthwise slices at the ends of the sweet potato; discard or save for another use.

3. In a medium bowl, coat the sweet potato with ½ teaspoon oil. Season with salt and pepper.

4. Arrange the sweet potato slices in a single layer on a foil-lined baking sheet and roast for 15 minutes. Flip and rotate, then return to the oven for 5 minutes. Remove and let cool for at least 5 minutes.

5. Meanwhile, make the dressing. Place the frozen raspberries, balsamic vinegar, 2 tablespoons oil, honey, chia seeds, salt, and pepper in a blender or food processor, or place in a bowl and use a hand blender. Blend until smooth. Makes about 6 tablespoons, so you'll have extra.

6. Assemble the "toasts." Top each with 1 tablespoon yogurt, drizzle with ½ teaspoon dressing, and garnish with a slice of persimmon, pomegranate arils, and thyme leaves.

Tip: *Shaped like small beefsteak tomatoes, Fuyu persimmon are seasonal. If they are not available, use apples or pears.*

Gimbap

Time: 30 to 60 minutes   **Makes:** 4 rolls

2 cups cooked brown rice

1 tablespoon toasted
sesame oil, divided

2 teaspoons olive oil, divided

2 eggs

1 tablespoon water

10 ounces baby spinach

4 sheets dried seaweed
sheets, about 8 x 10 inches

1 medium Quickle Rainbow
Carrots (page 156),
cut into thin strips

salt, to taste

1. Set aside a small spoonful of the cooked rice. In a medium
bowl, combine the remaining rice with salt and 2 teaspoons
sesame oil. Set aside.

2. Heat 1 teaspoon olive oil in a large nonstick pan over
medium heat until hot but not smoking. While the pan heats,
whisk the eggs with the water in a medium bowl. Pour into the
hot pan in a thin layer and cook for 60 to 90 seconds. Flip and
cook for another 30 to 60 seconds. Transfer to a cutting board,
let cool slightly, then slice into ¼-inch strips.

3. Add the remaining teaspoon olive oil to the pan if it seems
dry. Heat until hot but not smoking, then add the spinach and
gently stir until just wilted, about 2 minutes.

4. Transfer to a medium bowl, season with salt and 1 teaspoon
sesame oil. You should have about 1½ cups loosely packed
spinach. Once cool enough to handle, transfer to a fine-mesh
strainer and squeeze enough liquid to reduce the volume by
half, to about ¾ cup.

5. Lay a seaweed sheet, smooth shiny side down and rougher
dull side up, on a bamboo roller or parchment paper. Spread
½ cup rice on the seaweed so that it goes end-to-end the
longer way, but covers only two-thirds the shorter way. Lay a
quarter of the carrot, egg, and spinach in a flat row on the rice,

starting an inch or so from the rice end of the seaweed sheet. Roll starting from the rice end, keeping the roll tight as you go along. When you get close to the end, smear a few grains of the reserved rice across the top to act as glue. Use a few drops of water if the ends aren't sealing. Give the finished roll a final squeeze to ensure the contents are packed tightly. Cut into 10 to 12 pieces with a serrated knife. Repeat the process to make three more rolls.

Tip: *Wet your hands or a spatula to spread the rice so that it doesn't stick to you or your tools, and sticks only to the seaweed. The kind of seaweed that works best is sometimes called laver. It is drier and thicker than snacking seaweed, which is thin, oil-roasted and salted. You can try subbing other proteins and vegetables for variety.*

Quickle Rainbow Carrots

Time: 30 to 60 minutes **Serves:** 8

1¼ cups water

1 cup apple cider vinegar

4 sprigs fresh dill

½ teaspoon juniper berries, lightly crushed

2 bunches rainbow carrots

1. In a medium pot, make the pickling liquid by boiling the water with the vinegar, dill, and juniper berries until fragrant. Keep at a boil for 2 minutes, then let the liquid cool.

2. In a separate medium pot, fill halfway with water and bring to a boil. Meanwhile, prepare an ice bath.

3. Blanch the carrots in the boiling water until just softened, 1 to 2 minutes. Using a slotted spoon, transfer to the ice bath and gently agitate until cool, then drain and dry.

4. Slice the carrots into large matchsticks and place in a small shallow dish. Pour the cooled pickling liquid over the carrots, and let pickle for 30 minutes.

5. Serve immediately or refrigerate with the pickling liquid in an airtight container for up to 2 months.

Tip: *These quickles go great with a tart yogurt dip, hummus, or za'atar spice blend.*

Lemony Asparagus

Time: < 30 minutes   **Serves:** 2

1 teaspoon olive oil

1 pound thin asparagus spears

zest and juice from 1 lemon

1 teaspoon grated fresh ginger

2–3 tablespoons almond slices

1 teaspoon sesame oil

salt and pepper, to taste

1. In a large nonstick pan over medium heat, heat the olive oil until hot but not smoking. Add the asparagus and season to taste with salt and pepper. Stir frequently until crisp-tender, about 8 minutes.

2. Add most of the lemon zest along with the ginger, almonds, and lemon juice. Stir to combine until the lemon juice is slightly sticky, about 2 minutes.

3. Remove from the heat and serve with the remaining lemon zest and drizzle the sesame oil over top. Season with salt and pepper to taste.

Apple Wakame Seaweed Salad

Time: < 30 minutes   **Serves:** 4

2 ounces wakame seaweed

¼ cup rice vinegar

zest and juice from 1 lime

1 tablespoon soy sauce

1 tablespoon minced or grated ginger

1 teaspoon sugar

¼ cup avocado oil

1 teaspoon toasted sesame oil

1 medium apple, thinly sliced

toasted sesame seeds (optional)

salt and pepper, to taste

1. In a large bowl, cover the seaweed with cold water and let soak until softened, 5 to 10 minutes. Drain and squeeze out excess liquid, then roughly chop. Place back in the large bowl.

2. To make the dressing, whisk together the vinegar, lime zest and juice, soy sauce, ginger, sugar, avocado oil, and sesame oil in a medium bowl. Season with salt and pepper.

3. Pour the dressing over the seaweed, and massage with clean or gloved hands to combine. Fold in the apple slices. Taste and adjust seasoning if needed.

4. Serve immediately. Garnish with sesame seeds, if using.

Tip: A sweet, crisp, slightly tart apple works best in this recipe to offer contrasting texture and flavor. Try a Honey Crisp, Fuji, or Braeburn apple.

Garlicky Summer Squash

Time: < 30 minutes   **Serves:** 4

1 tablespoon olive oil

1 clove garlic, minced

1 medium zucchini, sliced into ½-inch rounds

1 medium yellow summer squash, sliced into ½-inch rounds

1 tablespoon chopped pistachios

salt and pepper, to taste

1. Heat the oil in a large nonstick pan over medium heat until hot but not smoking. Add the garlic and stir until fragrant, 20 to 30 seconds. Add the zucchini and summer squash, season with salt and pepper, and sauté until tender-crisp, 3 to 5 minutes.

2. Before serving, garnish with pistachios.

Roasted Delicata Squash

Time: < 30 minutes   **Serves:** 2

1 (6–8 inch) delicata squash

1 tablespoon olive oil,
plus more as needed

2 teaspoons sumac

1 teaspoon ground turmeric

½ teaspoon red chile flakes

½ teaspoon garlic powder

½ teaspoon onion powder

¼ teaspoon pepper

¼ teaspoon salt

1. Preheat the oven to 425°F.

2. Cut the squash in half lengthwise, scrape the seeds out with a spoon, then thinly slice into half rings, leaving the skin on (it's edible). In a large bowl, combine the half rings with the remaining ingredients.

3. On a large baking sheet lined with foil, arrange the seasoned half rings in a single layer. Roast for 5 to 7 minutes, rotate (drizzle with more olive oil if the squash looks dry), and roast for a final 5 to 7 minutes, or until fork tender.

Fig and Wheat Berry Grain Salad

Time: 1 to 2 hours **Serves:** 4

½ cup hazelnuts

2 cups cooked wheat berries

¼ cup Raspberry Vinaigrette (page 210), plus more as needed

4 cups baby arugula

12 fresh figs, quartered, or 8 dried figs, roughly chopped

4 sprigs fresh mint, leaves only, thinly sliced

4 sprigs fresh basil, leaves only, thinly sliced

1. Preheat the oven to 350°F.

2. Arrange the hazelnuts on a baking sheet and roast for 10 minutes, or until the hazelnuts smell nutty and are toasted. Set aside to cool.

3. In a large bowl, combine the wheat berries and the Raspberry Balsamic Vinaigrette, coating the grain well. Fold in the arugula, three-quarters of the figs, three-quarters of the hazelnuts, half the mint, and half the basil. Gently combine the ingredients, then transfer to a serving dish.

4. Garnish with the remaining figs, hazelnuts, and herbs. Serve with additional vinaigrette on the side.

Tip: *If you prefer, use farro or barley in place of the wheat berries. Carefully monitor the hazelnuts as they toast to avoid burning them. Roll the herbs to make it easier to thinly slice.*

Couscous with Grapes and Snow Peas

Time: < 30 minutes

3 teaspoons olive oil, divide

½ cup snow peas

1 cup water

1 cup uncooked whole wheat couscous

2 cups halved red grapes

salt and pepper, to taste

1. In a large nonstick skillet, heat 1 teaspoon olive oil over medium heat until hot but not smoking. Sauté the snow peas for 1 minute, and season with salt and pepper to taste. Remove from the pan and set aside.

2. Add the water to the pan and bring to a boil. Add the couscous, stirring well. Turn off the heat, cover, let stand 5 minutes, then fluff with a fork.

3. In a large bowl, gently combine the couscous, snow peas, grape halves, and 2 teaspoons olive oil. Season with salt and pepper to taste. Drizzle more olive oil before serving if desired.

Quinoa Asparagus Pistachio Salad

Time: 30 to 60 minutes   **Serves:** 4 to 6

2 cups uncooked rainbow quinoa

½ cup pistachios

1 teaspoon olive oil

16 thin asparagus spears, cut into 2-inch pieces

½ cup sliced green beans (2-inch pieces)

¾ cup French Vinaigrette (page 211)

2 tablespoons chopped fresh basil

2 tablespoons chopped fresh parsley

1 lemon, zested and quartered

1. Cook the quinoa according to package directions.

2. Heat a large nonstick pan over medium-low heat until warm. Add the pistachios and toast them, stirring frequently, 1 to 2 minutes or until they just begin to smell nutty and toasty. Remove from the heat and let cool.

3. In the same pan used for the pistachios, add oil and sauté asparagus and green beans until tender-crisp, 3–5 minutes.

4. In a large bowl, combine the cooked quinoa, asparagus, and green beans with the French Vinaigrette. Toss to coat.

5. Fold in the toasted pistachios along with the basil and parsley.

6. Garnish with lemon zest, and serve with lemon wedges on the side.

Coconut Curry Sorghum and Greens

Time: 1 to 2 hours   **Serves:** 4

Coconut Sorghum:

1 cup uncooked sorghum, rinsed

¾ cup coconut milk

2¼ cups almond milk

large pinch of salt

Curry:

1 tablespoon olive oil

1 medium sweet onion, chopped

6 cloves garlic, roughly chopped

1 tablespoon curry powder

1 teaspoon ground ginger

½ teaspoon chile powder

¾ cup coconut milk

2 cups almond milk

3 tablespoons rice wine vinegar or mirin

salt and pepper, to taste

Squash:

1 medium delicata squash

1 tablespoon olive oil

pinch of curry powder

salt and pepper, to taste

Base and Garnishes:

4 cups lightly packed baby spinach

1 (8-inch) cucumber, thinly sliced

2 tablespoons Marcona almonds

2–3 chives, finely chopped

10–15 fresh mint leaves, torn or cut into strips

red chile flakes (optional)

1. Preheat the oven to 375°F.

2. To make the coconut sorghum, combine the sorghum, coconut milk, almond milk, and salt in a large pot. Bring to a boil over medium-high heat, then lower to a simmer and cover for 50 to 60 minutes, or until cooked to desired consistency.

3. Meanwhile, make the curry. Heat the oil in a large nonstick saucepan over medium heat until hot but not smoking. Add the onion and stir occasionally until soft, about 3 minutes. Add the garlic and spices, and stir constantly for about 30 seconds or until fragrant. Add the coconut milk, almond milk, and rice wine vinegar or mirin, and bring to a boil, stirring occasionally. Lower the heat and simmer for about 30 minutes, or to desired consistency. Season with salt and pepper to taste.

4. While the coconut sorghum and curry simmer, make the squash. Lightly oil a medium foil-lined sheet pan. Cut the squash lengthwise and scrape out the seeds. Leaving the skin on, slice into 1-inch-thick half rings. In a large bowl, toss the half rings with the oil, curry powder, and salt and pepper. Arrange in a single layer on the sheet pan. Roast for 5 to 6 minutes on one side, flip, and return to the oven for another 5 to 6 minutes, or until a fork easily pierces the flesh. Remove from the oven and let cool 10 minutes.

5. To plate the dish either family style or divided evenly among 4 plates, make a bed of baby spinach, spoon the coconut sorghum over the greens, and top with the roasted squash. Drizzle the curry (serve any extra on the side). Garnish with cucumbers slices, almonds, chives, and mint. If using red chile flakes, sprinkle a pinch over the dish or serve on the side.

Tip: *One 13.5-ounce can of coconut milk is the perfect amount for this recipe—simply divide it between the coconut sorghum and curry recipes. Right after the dish is served, stir the warm ingredients so they'll wilt the spinach and infuse it with curry flavors.*

Poached Chicken and Buckwheat Soba Bowls

Time: 30 to 60 minutes   **Serves:** 4 to 6

1 pound boneless skinless chicken breasts

2 teaspoons olive oil

½ cup water

1 (8–9 ounce) package mugwort-buckwheat soba noodles

4–6 eggs (1 per person)

1 teaspoon sesame oil

2 tablespoons mirin

1 tablespoon unseasoned rice vinegar

1 tablespoon soy sauce

1 medium cucumber, sliced into rounds

black sesame seeds, sliced scallion greens (optional)

salt and pepper, to taste

Salsa Verde:

¾ cup loosely packed fresh mint leaves

3 cups loosely packed fresh flat-leaf parsley leaves

2 anchovy fillets

3 tablespoons capers

zest from 1 lemon

2 tablespoons red wine vinegar

½ cup extra-virgin olive oil

1. Pat dry the chicken breasts with paper towels, and season both sides with salt and pepper.

2. Heat a shallow pan over medium heat until hot. Add the olive oil and swirl. Add the chicken, breast side down, and cook for 5 minutes. Flip, pour in the water, and continue cooking until the chicken has cooked through and the water has cooked off, about 5 minutes. Remove to a cutting board and let rest until cool.

3. In a medium pot, heat water for the soba noodles. Cook according to package directions. Set aside.

4. In a medium pot over high heat, heat water for soft-boiled eggs. When the water is at a rolling boil, carefully add the eggs and cook for 5 to 7 minutes. Meanwhile, prepare an ice bath. When the eggs are done, transfer to the ice bath to stop the cooking process. Once cool, peel carefully and set aside.

5. In a small bowl, whisk to combine the sesame oil, mirin, rice vinegar, and soy sauce. Pour half over the noodles and toss to coat. Set aside.

6. Shred the chicken with a fork, and toss with the other half of the sauce. Set aside.

7. To make the salsa verde, pulse all ingredients in a food processor until finely chopped but not liquified. As an alternative, finely chop and stir together all the ingredients.

8. Plate the noodles in individual bowls, and top with the chicken and cucumber. To each bowl, add a peeled, whole egg topped with a generous spoonful of salsa verde. Garnish with black sesame seeds and scallions, if using.

Tip: *If chicken is thick, cut or pound to a uniform thickness of about 1 inch for even cooking. There may be extra salsa verde, which is delicious on just about anything—eggs, toast, poultry, fish.*

Turkey Stuffed Bell Peppers

Time: < 30 minutes   **Serves:** 2

2 medium yellow or orange bell peppers, cut in half lengthwise from stem to base

2 teaspoons olive oil

8 ounces ground turkey

1 teaspoon ground cumin

1 medium onion, chopped

½ cup canned black beans, drained and rinsed

½ cup canned roasted whole tomatoes, large dice, liquid reserved

2 sprigs fresh cilantro, chopped

Cashew Crema (page 213, optional)

salt and pepper, to taste

1. Turn on the broiler.

2. Place the bell peppers cut face down on a foil-lined baking sheet and broil. Check on them after 2 minutes, and broil for up to 5 minutes, until just softened but intact.

3. Make the stuffing. In a large nonstick pan over medium-high heat, heat the oil until hot but not smoking. Add the ground turkey and cumin, season with salt and pepper, and cook for 3 to 5 minutes, stirring and breaking the turkey into pieces. Add the onion and cook another 2 minutes, until just softened. Season again with salt and pepper. Add the beans and tomatoes, and cook until warmed through and the mixture becomes saucelike, about 2 minutes. Add some of the reserved tomato liquid if the mixture seems dry.

4. Stuff each of the 4 pepper "boats" with the filling. Serve any extra on the side. Garnish with cilantro and drizzle with Cashew Crema, if using.

Tip: *If you have any leftover thick sauce such as Roasted Carrot Spread with Herb Oil (page 208) or Red Beet Hummus (page 206), add a spoonful or two to the plate first to keep the bell pepper from sliding.*

Pistachio-Crusted Chicken

Time: 30 to 60 minutes   **Serves:** 2

1 pound boneless skinless chicken breasts

½ cup coarsely ground pistachios

zest from 1 lemon

2 teaspoons sumac

½ teaspoon salt

1 cup whole wheat flour

2 eggs

1 tablespoon water

salt and pepper, to taste

1. Preheat the oven to 400°F.

2. Pat dry the chicken breasts, cut into 1-inch-thick strips, and season with salt and pepper.

3. Place the pistachios, lemon zest, sumac, and salt in a small bowl. Stir to mix well, then transfer to a shallow plate.

4. Pour the flour onto another shallow plate.

5. In a medium bowl, whisk the eggs with the water.

6. Place a shallow wire rack on a large rimmed baking sheet lined with foil. Working with one chicken strip at a time, dredge the chicken in the flour, shake off the excess, dip in the beaten egg, let the excess drip off, and coat in the pistachio mixture. Transfer to the wire rack. Discard any remaining flour, pistachio mixture, and egg.

7. Bake the chicken strips for 15 to 20 minutes, or until the chicken is cooked through and the coating is crisp.

Tip: You can substitute precut chicken tenders for the chicken breasts and, for a gluten-free option, almond or coconut flour for the whole wheat flour. An instant-read thermometer can tell you if the chicken is cooked to a safe internal temperature of 165°F. The baking time may vary depending on the thickness of the chicken.

Taco Bowl

Time: 30 to 60 minutes   **Serves:** 2

½ cup uncooked brown rice

½ pound skinless chicken tenders, large dice

2 teaspoons chile powder

½ teaspoon ground cumin

¼ teaspoon salt

¼ teaspoon freshly ground pepper

1 tablespoon olive oil

½ small onion, diced

½ avocado, diced

1 lime, zested and quartered

1 cup canned black beans, drained and rinsed

½ cup fresh, canned, or cooked from frozen corn kernels

2 Roma tomatoes

Cashew Crema (page 213, optional)

2–4 sprigs fresh cilantro, roughly chopped

1. Cook the rice according to package instructions.

2. Pat dry the chicken with paper towels, and season with the chile powder, cumin, salt, and pepper.

3. Heat the oil in a large nonstick pan over medium-high heat until hot but not smoking. Cook the onion until just wilted and aromatic, 1 to 2 minutes. Add the spiced chicken and let cook for 1 minute undisturbed, then stir occasionally for another 3 to 5 minutes, or until just cooked through. Remove from the heat and set aside.

4. Place the diced avocado in a small bowl and squeeze the juice from two lime wedges over top to keep the avocado from browning.

5. Assemble the taco bowls. Divide the rice between two bowls. Top with the chicken, beans, corn, tomatoes, and avocado. Add a drizzle of Cashew Crema, if using. Garnish each bowl with cilantro and a lime wedge.

Tip: *For a change of pace, try substituting ground turkey for the chicken tenders, and quinoa for the brown rice.*

Spicy Lemongrass Poached Prawns

Time: 30 to 60 minutes   **Serves:** 4

1 stalk lemongrass, bottom
6 inches halved lengthwise
and thinly sliced, top mashed

½ bunch fresh cilantro,
leaves and stems separated

3 sprigs fresh mint, leaves
and stems separated

1 shallot, thinly sliced,
ends reserved

1 bird's-eye chile, thinly
sliced, ends reserved

1 pound prawns or colossal
shrimp (10–15 per pound),
shell-on, deveined

1 clove garlic, minced,
sprinkled with salt, mashed
with back of knife to
make a rough paste

2 tablespoons fish sauce

⅓ cup lime juice (about
2–3 limes), lime peels reserved

2 scallions, whites sliced,
greens sliced and reserved

1 head butter lettuce

½ inch fresh ginger, cut
into matchsticks

1. To a large pot of water, add the mashed lemongrass top, cilantro stems, mint stems, shallot and chile ends (include some discarded seeds, if desired), and lime peels. Place over high heat and bring to boil; cook at a boil for 15 minutes. Turn the heat off, add the prawns or colossal shrimp and cover for 3 minutes, or until opaque. Let cool, then peel and halve lengthwise.

2. Meanwhile, make the dressing. Combine the remaining lemongrass and chile with the garlic, fish sauce, lime juice, and white portion of scallions. Set aside.

3. Plate on a serving platter. Start with a bed of lettuce. Add all the ginger and most of the shallot slices, and cilantro and mint leaves. Dunk the shrimp in the dressing, shake off the excess, then place on top of the salad. Spoon the dressing over

the salad. Garnish with the scallion greens, and the remaining shallots slices and cilantro and mint leaves.

Tip: *This dish works well deconstructed—set up stations of lettuce, shrimp, herbs, shallots, ginger, scallions, and dressing, and let people fill their own lettuce cups. Bird's-eye chile is sometimes sold as Thai chile. If it's not available, serrano chile is a fine substitute. If the prawns do not come deveined, use kitchen shears to cut down the full length of prawn backs, then strip out the vein.*

Sheet Pan Salmon

Time: 30 to 60 minutes   **Serves:** 2

2 skin-on salmon fillets
(about 4 ounces each)

3 tablespoons olive
oil, divided

1 bunch broccoli

2 pinches of red chile
flakes (optional)

¼ cup roasted almonds,
roughly chopped

¼ cup sun-dried tomatoes,
roughly chopped

6–8 sprigs fresh mint,
roughly chopped

salt and pepper, to taste

1. Preheat the oven to 425°F. Line a sheet pan with foil.

2. Pat dry the salmon with paper towels. Season with salt and pepper. Place on one end of the sheet pan and drizzle with 1 tablespoon oil.

3. Trim all sides of the broccoli stalk, and cut the tender core into 1-inch pieces. Cut the broccoli florets into 1-inch pieces. In a medium bowl, toss with 1 tablespoon oil and 1 pinch of red chile flakes, if using. Season with salt and pepper to taste. Place on the other end of the sheet pan.

4. Roast for 5 minutes. Remove from the oven and give the broccoli a stir. Return to the oven to roast another 4 minutes.

5. Meanwhile, combine the almonds, sun-dried tomatoes, mint, 1 tablespoon oil, and 1 pinch of red chile flakes, if using. Season with salt and pepper to taste.

6. To serve, top the salmon with almond and tomato mixture.

Blackened Tilapia

Time: < 30 minutes   **Serves:** 4

2 teaspoons ground cumin

2 teaspoons paprika

2 teaspoons pepper

½ teaspoon salt

1 teaspoon coffee grounds

2 teaspoons dried oregano

4 (6-ounce) tilapia fillets

1 teaspoon olive oil,
plus more as needed

1 lemon, quartered

Salsa:

1 medium ripe
avocado, cubed

1 medium mango, cubed

⅓ cup finely chopped
red onion

2 tablespoons minced
fresh cilantro

juice of 1 lime

salt and pepper, to taste

1. In a small bowl, combine the cumin, paprika, pepper, salt, coffee, and oregano. On a large plate, pat dry the fish with paper towels. Rub the spice mixture onto both sides of the fish. Let rest for 15 to 30 minutes.

2. To make the salsa, stir together all the ingredients in a medium bowl. Cover and refrigerate until ready to use. It can be made a day ahead.

3. In a large nonstick pan, heat 1 teaspoon oil over medium heat until hot but not smoking. Working in batches if necessary, cook the fish for 2 to 4 minutes per side until opaque and cooked through. Transfer to a plate to cool. Add more oil between batches if the pan is dry.

4. To serve, garnish each filet with a spoonful of salsa and a lemon wedge. Serve the remaining salsa on the side.

Tip: *You can use catfish or another white fish in place of the tilapia.*

Spaghetti alle Vongole

Time: < 30 minutes   **Serves:** 2

2 pounds littleneck clams	¼ cup white wine
6 ounces whole grain spaghetti	¼ cup pistachios, crushed, divided
3 tablespoons olive oil, plus more as needed	2 tablespoons chopped fresh flat-leaf parsley, divided
2 cloves garlic, thinly sliced	cornmeal (optional)
¼ teaspoon gochugaru or red chile flakes	salt and pepper, to taste

1. Prepare three large bowls of cold water with a generous pinch of salt or cornmeal to help the clams release any grit inside. Soak the clams in the first bowl for 20 minutes. Transfer to the second bowl for another 20 minutes. Transfer one last time to the third bowl for a final 20 minutes. Scrub the outside of the clams and store uncovered on ice until ready to use.

2. Prepare the spaghetti according to package instructions, but remove a couple of minutes early, before it's al dente. Reserve ½ cup cooking liquid before draining.

3. In a large nonstick skillet, heat the oil over medium heat until hot but not smoking. Add the garlic, and stir constantly until fragrant and just starting to turn color. Add the gochugaru or red chile flakes and cook another 15 seconds. Add the wine and clams, and turn the heat to high. Cover and cook until the clams open, about 3 to 6 minutes.

4. Add half the reserved pasta water to the skillet and bring to a boil. Add the spaghetti and finish cooking to al dente, tossing to coat with the sauce, about 2 minutes. Add more pasta water if the sauce seems too thick or dry. Turn off the heat. Fold in most of the crushed pistachios and half the parsley. Season with salt and pepper to taste.

5. Divide between two bowls. Garnish with the remaining pistachios and parsley and a drizzle of olive oil.

Tip: *Examine the clams before using them. If a clam is open and you tap it closed, it should react. If it doesn't react and stays open, toss it out as that means it has died.*

Harissa-Spiced Striped Bass

Time: 30 to 60 minutes   **Serves:** 4

1 pound striped bass

1½ tablespoons harissa

1 medium orange

1 medium lemon

1 pound purple
potatoes, quartered

1½ pounds brussels
sprouts, halved

3 tablespoons olive
oil, divided

1 cup water

1 cup uncooked whole
wheat couscous

1 shallot, thinly sliced

1 pint cherry tomatoes, halved

3 sprigs fresh parsley, chopped

salt and pepper, to taste

1. Preheat the oven to 425°F.

2. Pat dry the bass with paper towels and season with salt and harissa. Cut three thin slices of orange starting from the center, and five thin slices of lemon starting from the center. Arrange the orange and lemon slices on top of fish. Reserve the citrus end pieces.

3. In a large bowl, toss the potatoes and brussels sprouts with 2 tablespoons olive oil and salt and pepper. Arrange in one layer on a large sheet pan lined with foil. Roast for 10 minutes. Remove from the oven, add the seasoned bass and roast for another 12 minutes, or until the fish is fully cooked. Remove from the oven and let rest.

4. While the fish is cooking, bring the water to a boil in a medium pot. Turn the heat off, add the couscous, cover, and let stand 5 minutes, then fluff with a fork.

5. To make the tomato salad, squeeze the juice from the remaining orange ends into a small bowl. Add the shallot, tomatoes, parsley, and 1 tablespoon olive oil, and season with salt and pepper to taste.

6. To serve, spoon tomato salad on top of the fish, or serve on the side. Serve the couscous on the side along with four mini lemon wedges cut from the remainder of the lemon.

Tip: *To get a nice char on the brussels sprouts, roast cut side down. To keep the purple of the potatoes vibrant, roast cut side up.*

Ratatouille

Time: 1 to 2 hours   **Serves:** 4 to 6

1 medium eggplant, thinly sliced

3 Roma tomatoes, thinly sliced

1 large yellow summer squash, thinly sliced

1 large zucchini, thinly sliced

3 small red potatoes, thinly sliced

3 yellow and orange mini sweet peppers, thinly sliced

6 tablespoons olive oil, divided, plus more as needed

6 cloves garlic, chopped

1 medium onion or shallot, chopped

1 (6-ounce) can tomato paste

1 tablespoon gochugaru or red chile flakes

1 (16-ounce) can fire-roasted crushed tomatoes

1 teaspoon fresh thyme leaves, divided

salt and pepper, to taste

1. Preheat the oven to 375°F.

2. Cut parchment paper to fit inside an oven-safe, heavy-bottomed pot 8 to 10 inches in diameter (this recipe was tested with a 9½-inch-diameter Dutch oven). You can trace the top of the pot or the lid, then cut a ¼ inch inside the line to get approximately the right size.

3. Arrange the slices of eggplant, tomato, summer squash, zucchini, potato, and sweet pepper in separate rows on a large sheet tray. Set aside.

4. In the pot, heat 3 tablespoons oil over medium heat until hot but not smoking. Add the garlic and onion or shallot and sauté until fragrant, 30 to 60 seconds. Add the tomato paste and gochugaru or red chile flakes, and stir to combine well. Heat until the tomato paste starts to darken.

5. Add the crushed tomatoes and half the thyme, stir to combine, and season with salt and pepper. Simmer until the sauce begins to thicken. If it's too thick, add a little water. It should be slightly thicker than pasta sauce, verging on jammy. Remove from the heat.

6. Starting from the outside in, lay the vegetable slices in concentric circles. It's easiest to create stacks, then place the stacks in the pot rather than arrange one slice at a time. One stack equals one slice of each vegetable. Place along the outer edge of the pot. Repeat until you've reached the center. If you have leftover vegetables, refrigerate for another use.

7. Drizzle the remaining 3 tablespoons olive oil over the dish, and season with salt and pepper to taste. Cover with parchment paper and bake for 55 minutes.

8. Remove from the oven, discard the parchment paper, and garnish with the remaining thyme leaves. Drizzle additional olive oil in the pot or on each plate. Season to taste.

Tip: Choose vegetables of about the same diameter to make them easy to stack. Instead of canned tomatoes, you can use 2 cups of your favorite jarred marinara sauce. The dish goes well with whole grain country bread or on top of whole wheat couscous.

Chickpea-Stuffed Sweet Potatoes

Time: 30 to 60 minutes   **Serves:** 2

2 medium sweet potatoes

1 cup canned chickpeas, drained and rinsed

1 teaspoon extra-virgin olive oil, divided

Yogurt Sauce:

1 small clove garlic

1 lemon

½ cup Greek yogurt

1 teaspoon ground cumin

4 sprigs fresh cilantro, leaves only, roughly chopped

4 sprigs fresh mint, leaves only, torn

¼ teaspoon curry powder

½ teaspoon extra-virgin olive oil

salt and pepper, to taste

1. Preheat the oven to 425°F.

2. Poke steam holes in the sweet potatoes and place on a baking sheet lined with foil. Bake for 40 to 50 minutes, or until fork tender. Remove from the oven and let cool slightly before handling.

3. In a medium bowl, combine the chickpeas, ½ teaspoon oil, cumin, and salt and pepper to taste. Toss to coat.

4. Heat ½ teaspoon oil in a nonstick pan over medium heat until hot but not smoking. Add the spiced chickpeas and shake the pan occasionally to stir. Cook until warmed through and fragrant, 3 to 5 minutes. Remove from the heat and set aside.

5. To make the yogurt sauce, mince the garlic, sprinkling a little salt on top to help it break down, then mashing with the back of a chef's knife to make a paste. Zest the lemon, mincing half and keeping half for garnish, then cut the lemon in half, juice half, and cut the other half into wedges. In a medium bowl, combine the yogurt, 1 teaspoon lemon juice, minced lemon zest, garlic paste, curry powder, and olive oil. Stir well. Season with salt and pepper to taste, or additional lemon juice if there is extra. Refrigerate until ready to serve.

6. To serve, carefully cut a lengthwise seam across the top of each sweet potato. Using two forks, gently wedge the potato open a little to make room for the chickpeas. Scoop out some of the flesh if desired. Top with a dollop of yogurt sauce and serve any remaining sauce on the side. Garnish with cilantro, mint, and remaining lemon zest, and serve any remaining herbs on the side. Place a lemon wedge on each plate.

Pulse Pasta Alfredo

Time: 30 to 60 minutes   **Serves:** 4

½ pound whole wheat pasta

2 tablespoons olive oil

1 pound cremini mushrooms, sliced

2 cloves garlic, sliced

1 tablespoon sweet vermouth

½ cup broth or stock

1 cup fresh peas

½ cup Cashew Crema (page 213)

2–3 sprigs fresh flat-leaf parsley, leaves only, roughly chopped

Plant-Based Parmesan (page 212)

1 teaspoon gochugaru or red chile flakes, plus more as needed

salt and pepper, to taste

1. Cook the pasta according to package instructions for an al dente result.

2. In a large nonstick skillet, heat the oil over medium heat until hot but not smoking. Add the mushrooms and garlic, and stir to coat. Season with salt and pepper. Stir occasionally until the mushrooms begin to reduce, about 5 minutes. Add the vermouth and stir to combine, then let cook, stirring only occasionally, until the mushrooms and liquid reduce further, about another 5 minutes.

3. To the same skillet, add the broth or stock and boil for 3 minutes, then stir in the peas to warm through, about 90 seconds. Turn off the heat. Add the cooked pasta, and Cashew Crema to the skillet and stir to combine. Season with salt and pepper to taste.

4. Serve in individual bowls or on plates. Garnish with parsley and gochugaru or red chile flakes, and serve Plant-Based Parmesan and additional gochugaru or red chile flakes on the side.

Tip: *This recipe offers many opportunities for substitutions. You can opt for chickpea, lentil, or quinoa pasta instead of whole wheat. Try substituting white button or shiitake mushrooms for the creminis (also called baby portobellos), or use all three. Instead of vermouth, go with cooking wine or additional broth or stock. If fresh peas aren't available, use frozen.*

Sorghum-Stuffed Butternut Squash

Time: 1 to 2 hours   **Serves:** 8

1 cup uncooked sorghum

2–3 cups chicken broth or stock, and more as needed

2 medium (about 2 pounds each) butternut squashes, halved lengthwise, seeds removed

4 tablespoons plus 1 teaspoon extra-virgin olive oil, divided

2 lemons

1 tablespoon champagne vinegar

3 tablespoons chopped dried figs, divided

½ medium red onion or 1 shallot, diced, divided

2 cloves garlic, minced

1 teaspoon chile flakes

1 cup canned chickpeas, drained and rinsed

7 cups baby spinach

salt and pepper, to taste

1. Preheat the oven to 375°F.

2. Cook the sorghum according to package directions, but using chicken stock or broth as your cooking liquid.

3. Meanwhile, place the squash halves cut side up on a sheet pan lined with foil. Brush all four cut sides with 1 tablespoon oil. Season with salt and pepper to taste. Roast in the oven for 45 minutes, then let rest until cool enough to handle.

4. Zest one lemon. Juice about 1½ lemons, or until you have 3 tablespoons of lemon juice. Reserve remaining lemon for another use.

5. To make the dressing, whisk 3 tablespoons oil, champagne vinegar, lemon juice, 1 tablespoon dried figs, 1 tablespoon red onion or shallot, one minced garlic clove, and salt and pepper. Makes about 4 ounces. Set aside.

6. In a large nonstick pan, heat 1 teaspoon olive oil over medium heat until hot but not smoking. Add the remaining red onion or shallot and sauté until just fragrant, about 30 seconds, then add the other minced garlic clove, and stir for another 30 seconds. Add 2 tablespoons dried figs and the chile flakes, and cook for 1 minute. Stir in the chickpeas and spinach, and cook for 3 to 4 minutes, or until spinach is just wilted. Turn off the heat, and stir in the lemon zest.

7. In a large bowl, combine the red onion or shallot mixture with the cooked sorghum. Pour in the dressing and toss to coat. Set aside.

8. Scoop out the center of each butternut squash half, leaving a ½- to 1-inch border. Spoon the filling evenly into the squash halves. Bake until heated through, about 10 minutes.

9. Serve warm. Sprinkle with pomegranate arils just before serving.

Tip: *Save the scooped squash flesh and add it to oatmeal, pancakes, smoothies, or soups. This dish tastes even better the next day, so count on leftovers.*

Buckwheat Spring Noodles

Time: 30 to 60 minutes   **Serves:** 4 to 6

1 large carrot, sliced into thin matchsticks

1 cup sugar snap peas

1 cup frozen shelled edamame

¼ cup rice wine vinegar or mirin

2 tablespoons soy sauce

2 tablespoons sesame oil, plus more as needed

2 teaspoons honey

½ inch fresh ginger, minced

1 clove garlic, minced

2 bundles buckwheat soba noodles (2 servings according to packaging)

2 teaspoons grapeseed or peanut oil

1 scallion, thinly sliced, white and green parts separated

½ cup kimchi, roughly chopped

sesame seeds, nori strips, soft-boiled eggs (optional)

1. Bring a large pot of water to a boil, and prepare an ice bath.

2. Blanch the carrots in the boiling water until just wilted, about 1 minute. Using a slotted spoon, transfer to the ice bath and agitate gently until cool. Drain and dry, then place in a large bowl.

3. Bring the water back to a boil and blanch the snap peas until bright green and still crisp, 1 to 2 minutes. As with the carrots, transfer to the ice bath, agitate until cool, drain, and dry. Slice in half on the diagonal, then add to the large bowl.

4. Bring the water back to a boil, add the edamame, and cook for 5 minutes, until just tender. As with the carrots and snap peas, transfer to the ice bath, agitate until cool, drain, and dry. Place in a medium bowl and combine with the rice wine vinegar or mirin, soy sauce, sesame oil, honey, ginger, and garlic. Toss to coat.

5. Bring the water back to a boil, add the soba noodles and cook until just tender, 2 to 3 minutes. Drain and rinse with cold water. Drain well, then add to the large bowl. Add sesame oil if mixture seems dry.

6. In a wok or large nonstick skillet, heat the grapeseed or peanut oil over medium heat until hot but not smoking. Add the white scallion parts, sauté until fragrant, about 1 minute. Add the edamame and marinade, and sauté until heated through, about 2 to 3 minutes. Transfer to the large bowl. Add the kimchi to the large bowl, and toss to combine.

7. Divide among two large bowls or plates, and garnish with the scallion greens, and sesame seeds, nori strips, or soft-boiled eggs, if using.

Walnut Lettuce Wraps

Time: < 30 minutes   **Serves:** 2

½ cup chopped carrots

½ cup chopped radishes

2 tablespoons rice vinegar

2 teaspoons gochugaru or red chile flakes, divided

1 cup chopped walnuts

1 tablespoon soy sauce

1 scallion, sliced, green and white parts separated

1 cup cooked brown rice

1 teaspoon toasted sesame oil

20 perilla leaves (optional)

1 head red leaf lettuce, about 20 or more leaves

1. In a medium bowl, combine the carrots and radishes with the rice vinegar and 1 teaspoon gochugaru or red chile flakes. Let soak for at least 10 minutes, stirring occasionally.

2. In a large nonstick pan over medium heat, sauté the walnuts for 1 to 2 minutes, stirring frequently. Lower the heat as soon as the nuts start to smell toasty. Add the soy sauce, white part of the scallion, and 1 teaspoon gochugaru or red chile flakes, and cook 1 to 2 minutes, stirring frequently. Remove from the heat and let cool in a large bowl.

3. In a medium bowl, combine the rice and sesame oil. Set aside.

4. With a slotted spoon, transfer the seasoned carrots and radishes to the bowl with the walnuts, and toss to combine.

5. Lay a perilla leaf, if using, inside each lettuce leaf. Divide the rice evenly among lettuce cups, top with the walnut mixture, and garnish with the green part of the scallion.

Tip: You can substitute liquid aminos for the soy sauce, and quinoa, barley, or sorghum for the brown rice. To up the veggie content and add another fresh note, slice a cucumber and add it on top of the walnut mixture.

Matcha-Ginger Chia Pudding

Time: < 30 minutes   **Serves:** 2

¼ cup black chia seeds

1 cup unsweetened vanilla almond-coconut milk

1½ tablespoons ginger syrup

1 teaspoon matcha powder

2–4 mint leaves

1. Whisk the chia seeds, almond-coconut milk, ginger syrup, and matcha powder together in a medium bowl. Let sit for at least 5 to 10 minutes so the chia seeds can soak.

2. Divide between two dessert cups, garnish with mint leaves, and enjoy immediately or cover and chill for 30 minutes or more before serving. This can be covered and stored in the refrigerator for up to 5 days.

Balsamic-Fig Nice Cream

Time: < 30 minutes (plus freezing time)   **Serves:** 2 to 4 (makes about 2 cups)

8 fresh Black Mission figs

1 teaspoon vanilla extract

1 teaspoon balsamic vinegar

½ cup unsweetened vanilla almond-coconut milk

2–8 mint leaves (optional)

1. In a high-powered blender or food processor, puree the figs and freeze in an ice cube tray for at least 2 hours.

2. Place the frozen figs along with the vanilla and balsamic vinegar in a blender or food processor, and pulse until combined but still semisolid. Add the almond-coconut milk slowly until desired consistency is reached.

3. To serve, scoop into individual dessert bowls, and garnish with mint leaves.

Tip: *You can use 1½ cups of your favorite frozen berries in place of figs.*

Spiced ABC Pudding (Avocado-Banana-Cocoa)

Time: < 30 minutes plus chilling time   **Serves:** 4 to 8

2 ripe medium avocados, roughly chopped

3 ripe medium bananas, roughly chopped

½ cup unsweetened cocoa powder

1 teaspoon vanilla extract

¼ teaspoon chile powder, plus more as needed

½ cup pistachios

zest from 1 medium orange

1. Preheat the oven to 350°F.

2. Place the avocados, bananas, cocoa, vanilla, and ¼ teaspoon chile powder in a blender, and blend until smooth. Cover and refrigerate for 1 to 2 hours, or until completely chilled.

3. Spread the pistachios on a baking sheet, and place in the oven for 3 minutes. Toss, and bake for an additional 3 minutes. Let cool and coarsely chop. Store in an airtight container until ready to serve.

4. To serve, spoon the pudding into individual dessert bowls, and top with the pistachios. Sprinkle the orange zest and chile powder, if desired, over top.

Dark Chocolate Bark

Time: > 2 hours (plus chilling time)   **Serves:** 6

8 ounces dark chocolate
(about 70%)

¼ teaspoon cinnamon

¼ teaspoon chile powder

¼ cup chopped pistachios,
almonds, or walnuts

¼ cup thinly sliced,
seeded kumquats

flaky salt (optional)

1. Fill a medium pot with water to about a quarter full and bring to a simmer.

2. Meanwhile, line a large rimmed baking sheet with parchment paper.

3. Place a large heat-resistant bowl over the pot of simmering water. The bottom of the bowl should be partially in the pot, but not touching the water. Or use a double boiler if you have one.

4. Place the chocolate, cinnamon, and chile powder in the bowl, and stir occasionally until the chocolate has melted. It should be approximately the temperature of your lips, so give it a taste. Pour the mixture in an even layer on the lined baking sheet. Tap the baking sheet or use a spatula to help spread the chocolate.

5. Quickly add the nuts and kumquat slices. Use plastic gloves or clean hands to lightly press the toppings into the chocolate. Garnish with flaky salt, if using.

6. Let cool at room temperature until completely hardened, at least 2 hours. The bark will harden in the refrigerator in about 15 minutes but may show condensation.

7. Peel the parchment paper away and break into bite-size pieces. Serve immediately, or refrigerate in an airtight container for up to 3 days.

Tip: *If you can't find or don't like kumquats, try orange zest instead. For shelf life up to a week at room temperature, use only dried fruit and nuts that don't need refrigeration.*

Banana Bread Trifle

Time: 1 to 2 hours   **Serves:** 4

Banana Bread:

2½ cups sliced overripe bananas (about 3–4 large bananas)

¼ cup olive oil

2 eggs

1 tablespoon vanilla extract

½ cup Greek yogurt

2 cups whole wheat pastry flour

1 teaspoon baking soda

½ teaspoon baking powder

½ teaspoon salt

½ cup chopped walnuts

Trifle:

4 cups 1-inch cubes loosely packed banana bread (see above)

8 ounces pomegranate juice

4 cups Greek yogurt

1 teaspoon vanilla extract

1 tablespoon honey

¼ teaspoon cardamom

2 cups blueberries (about 12 ounces)

2 cups sliced strawberries (about 16 ounces)

To make the Banana Bread:

1. Preheat the oven to 400°F. Grease a 4 x 8-inch loaf pan.

2. On a sheet pan lined with foil, arrange banana slices in a single layer and roast for 15 minutes. Remove from the oven and let cool. Lower the heat to 325°F.

3. In a large bowl, combine the roasted banana slices with the oil, eggs, vanilla, and yogurt until smooth.

4. In a medium bowl, combine the flour, baking soda, baking powder, and salt.

5. Sift the dry ingredients into the wet ingredients, using a spoon to break up any clumps, and stir to combine.

6. Fold the walnuts into the batter, then pour into the greased loaf pan. Bake for 45 minutes, or until a toothpick comes out clean. Set aside to cool.

To assemble the Trifle:

1. Once the banana bread is cool, cut into cubes and arrange in a single layer in a baking dish. Pour the pomegranate juice over top and let it soak into the bread.

2. In a medium bowl, combine the yogurt, vanilla, honey, and cardamom. Set aside.

3. Reserve a few blueberries and strawberries for garnish.

4. If using one serving dish, choose a large clear bowl and layer half the banana bread, half of the strawberries, a third of the yogurt, the blueberries, a third of the yogurt, the other half of the banana bread, the other half of the strawberries, and top with the final third of yogurt. Garnish with the reserved berries.

5. If using four 2-cup mason jars, in each jar layer ¼ cup banana bread, ¼ cup strawberries, ⅓ cup yogurt, ½ cup blueberries, ⅓ cup yogurt, ¼ cup banana bread, ¼ cup strawberries, and ⅓ cup yogurt. Garnish with the reserved berries.

Tip: To speed up banana ripening, place the bananas and an apple in a brown paper bag for a few days. Bake the bread a day ahead, and assembly becomes a snap the next day. Put the yogurt in a plastic food bag, then snip the bottom corner to make a piping bag. No sifter? Use a whisk to break up clumps in the dry ingredients. If you have blackberries and raspberries on hand, you can substitute them for the blueberries and strawberries.

Spiced Cider

Time: 1 to 2 hours   **Serves:** 4

4 cups pomegranate juice

zest and juice from
1 small orange

1 cup water

4 cinnamon sticks, plus
more as needed

6 whole cloves

1 pod star anise

6 pods green cardamom

6 juniper berries

1½ teaspoons vanilla extract

orange slices (optional)

1. Combine the pomegranate juice, orange juice and zest, water, cinnamon, cloves, star anise, cardamom, juniper berries, and vanilla in a large pot over medium heat and bring to a simmer. Lower the heat to keep simmering uncovered for 45 minutes.

2. Remove from the heat and let the flavors combine for 2 hours. Strain and garnish with orange zest along with extra cinnamon sticks and orange slices, if using. Refrigerate any leftovers, and reheat to serve.

Chai Latte

Time: < 30 minutes   **Serves:** 2

1½ cups water

2 teaspoons loose-leaf black tea or 2 tea bags black tea

1½ cups unsweetened vanilla almond-coconut milk, divided

4 teaspoons arrowroot powder

2 teaspoons chai spice blend (see below)

¼ cup almond butter

honey or maple syrup (optional)

Spice Blend:

1½ teaspoons ground ginger

1½ teaspoons ground cinnamon

½ teaspoon ground cloves

½ teaspoon ground nutmeg

½ teaspoon ground cardamom

½ teaspoon freshly ground pepper

1 pod star anise

1. In a small saucepan over high heat, bring the water to a boil, then remove from the heat. Once the water is calm and bubbles have subsided, add the tea and steep for 3 to 5 minutes. If using loose-leaf tea, strain and discard the tea leaves.

2. Whisk together ½ cup almond-coconut milk with the arrowroot powder until dissolved. Set aside.

3. In a small saucepan over medium-low heat, whisk together 1 cup almond-coconut milk, and the Spice Blend until well combined. Bring to a simmer, stirring occasionally.

4. Whisk in the mixture of almond-coconut milk and arrowroot until the liquid thickens, about 30 seconds. Remove from the heat immediately. Whisk in the black tea and almond butter until smooth.

5. Divide between two mugs. Add a drizzle of honey or maple syrup, if using.

Moon Milk

Time: < 30 minutes   **Serves:** 2

2½ cups unsweetened vanilla almond-coconut milk

1 teaspoon ground cardamom

1 teaspoon ground turmeric

1 teaspoon rose water

¼ teaspoon freshly ground pepper

1 teaspoon organic raw honey

crushed dried rose petals, cacao nibs, sesame seeds, chopped almonds, cardamom, turmeric (optional)

1. Combine all ingredients except the optional garnishes in a medium saucepan over medium-low heat, and gradually bring to a simmer, whisking periodically. Let simmer 1 minute, then remove from heat.

2. Divide between two mugs. Add one or more garnishes, if using.

Tip: *This beverage may also be known as a "turmeric latte" or "Golden Milk."*

Matcha Pomegranate Spritz

Time: < 30 minutes   **Serves:** 2

1 teaspoon matcha green tea powder

6–8 ounces steaming filtered water

8 ounces pomegranate juice

4–8 ounces sparkling water

1 lime, sliced into rounds

2 sprigs fresh mint

1. Fill a medium bowl with matcha powder and 6 to 8 ounces of steaming water. Use a whisk or frother to blend until matcha forms a top foam, about 1 to 2 minutes. Let cool.

2. To serve, add ice to two glasses, then evenly divide the pomegranate juice and matcha green tea. Top each glass with sparkling water, a slice of lime, and a mint sprig.

Turmeric Shot

Time: < 30 minutes   **Serves:** 2

Juice from a medium orange

1 tablespoon raw apple cider vinegar

¼ teaspoon ground turmeric

pinch of freshly ground pepper

1. Pour the juice in a small bowl and stir in the apple cider vinegar, turmeric, and pepper.

2. Serve chilled or over ice in two small glasses.

Virgin Sangria

Time: < 30 minutes plus chilling time   **Serves:** 8

1 inch fresh ginger, roughly chopped and mashed into a paste

1 ripe nectarine, sliced

1 ripe plum, sliced

1 orange, sliced

1 apple, peeled and chopped

2 cups Concord grape juice

2 cups pomegranate juice

juice of 1 lemon

juice of 1 lime

sparkling water

1. Place the mashed ginger in a large pitcher, then arrange the cut fruit in layers, reserving some pieces for garnish.

2. Pour the grape, pomegranate, lemon, and lime juices into the pitcher over the fruit, and stir gently with a long-handled spoon.

3. Cover and refrigerate for at least 3 hours, preferably overnight.

4. Stir before serving. To serve, start with a glass of ice, pour in ½ cup of the drink, add reserved fruit, and top off with sparkling water.

Coffee Banana Shake

Time: < 30 minutes   **Serves:** 2

2 frozen bananas

⅓ cup espresso or
½ cup strong coffee

¾ cup unsweetened vanilla
almond-coconut milk

1 tablespoon cocoa powder

1 tablespoon dark maple syrup
or manuka honey (optional)

Combine all ingredients in a high-powered blender until smooth, about 1 minute. Divide between two glasses. Makes about 20 ounces total.

Tip: Make sure the bananas are ripe before you freeze them. Peel and break a banana into two or three pieces before storing in the freezer.

Wild Slushie

Time: < 30 minutes   **Serves:** 2

1½ cups ice cubes

½ cup frozen wild blueberries

½ cup frozen tart cherries

2 tablespoons fresh lime juice

2–4 mint leaves

1. Combine all ingredients except the mint leaves in a high-powered blender, and blend until desired slushy consistency is reached.

2. Divide between two glasses and garnish with mint leaves. Serve immediately.

Magic Spicy Green Sauce

Time: <30 minutes   **Makes:** about 1½ cups

1 bunch fresh basil	1 clove garlic
1 bunch fresh cilantro	1 small jalapeño pepper
1 bunch fresh mint, leaves only	¼ cup olive oil
zest and juice of 1 lime	salt, pepper, and red chile flakes, to taste

Place all the ingredients except the oil in a food processor, and blend. Slowly drizzle in oil until the sauce is smooth or to desired consistency. Taste and adjust the seasoning if needed. Use immediately, store in an airtight container in the refrigerator for up to 3 days, or freeze for up to 4 months.

Tip: *Use as much of the jalapeño pepper as you like depending on your spice preference. If the sauce is too thick, thin it out with additional oil or lime juice. The sauce is delicious over eggs, on Avocado Toast (page 121), or on top of seafood and chicken.*

Gremolata

Time: < 30 minutes **Makes:** about ½ cup

zest and juice of 1 lemon

½ cup finely chopped
fresh parsley leaves

2 teaspoons finely
minced garlic

¼ teaspoon kosher salt

¼ teaspoon freshly
ground pepper

½ teaspoon gochugaru
or red chile flakes

In a small bowl, stir together all the ingredients. Use
immediately, store in an airtight container in the refrigerator for
up to 3 days, or freeze for up to 4 months.

*Tip: This sauce is delicious on Avocado Toast (page 121), seafood, or
sautéed vegetables.*

Red Beet Hummus

Time: < 30 minutes   **Makes:** 1½ to 2 cups

1 medium beet, quartered

¼ cup water

½ cup canned butter beans, drained and rinsed

2 cloves garlic

1 teaspoon sesame sauce

juice and zest of 1 lemon

salt, to taste

2 tablespoons olive oil, more as needed

sesame seeds (optional)

1. Place the beet in a medium microwave-safe bowl with the water and microwave for 3 to 5 minutes, until fork tender. Drain.

2. Place the microwaved beet in a food processor with the butter beans, garlic, sesame sauce, lemon juice and zest. Blend until smooth or to desired consistency. Season with salt to taste.

3. Garnish with olive oil and sesame seeds, if using. Use immediately, store in an airtight container in the refrigerator for up to 3 days, or freeze for up to 4 months.

Tip: *Serve this hummus with crudités, use as a sandwich spread, or smear on a plate under chicken, fish, or wilted greens. Tahini is one kind of sesame sauce.*

Pea Pistou

Time: <30 minutes   **Makes:** about 1 cup

½ cup frozen peas

1 bunch fresh flat-leaf parsley

zest and juice of ½ lemon

2 cloves garlic

¼ cup olive oil, plus more as needed

salt and pepper, to taste

In a food processor, blend all the ingredients until smooth or to desired consistency. Add more oil if the mixture is too thick. Use immediately, store in an airtight container in the refrigerator for up to 3 days, or freeze for up to 4 months.

Za'atar

Time: < 30 minutes   **Makes:** ½ cup

2 tablespoons fresh thyme leaves, minced

2 tablespoons toasted sesame seeds

2 teaspoons sumac

½ teaspoon coarse salt

Stir all the ingredients until well combined.

Tip: Although za'atar is traditionally made with ground sumac, you can substitute minced lemon zest. This blend goes great on top of thick yogurt such as Greek yogurt or Icelandic skyr and also works well as a garnish for hummus. Use immediately, store in an airtight container in the refrigerator for up to 3 days, or freeze for up to 4 months.

Roasted Carrot Spread with Herb Oil

Time: < 30 minutes   **Makes:** 2 cups spread and ¾ cup herb oil

4 medium carrots, cut into 2-inch pieces (about 2 cups)

¾ cup plus 1 teaspoon extra-virgin olive oil, divided, plus more as needed

1 bunch fresh cilantro or parsley (2–3 cups)

1 (15-ounce) can butter beans, drained and rinsed

1 clove garlic, smashed

juice of 1 lemon, plus more as needed

zest of juiced lemon (optional)

1 teaspoon sesame sauce

lemon wedges, radishes, toasted sesame seeds (optional)

salt and pepper, to taste

1. Preheat the oven to 400°F.

2. Toss the carrots with 1 teaspoon olive oil and salt and pepper to taste, then spread on a sheet pan lined with foil. Roast for 20 minutes.

2. To make an herb oil, combine the cilantro or parsley and ½ cup olive oil in a blender or food processor, and blend until smooth. Transfer to a bowl and set aside.

3. In the clean bowl of the blender or food processor, combine the roasted carrots, butter beans, garlic, lemon juice, half of the lemon zest if using, and sesame sauce. Drizzle in ¼ cup olive oil plus more as needed until the mixture is smooth or to desired consistency. Taste and adjust the seasoning if needed.

4. Place the spread in a bowl, and pour the desired amount of herb oil on one side. If using garnishes, arrange a few lemon wedges and radishes in the bowl and sprinkle a pinch of sesame seeds and the remaining lemon zest. Squeeze a little more lemon juice over top. Use immediately, or store in an airtight container in the refrigerator for up to 3 days. Freezing is not recommended.

Tip: *This spread is delectable with crudités, in whole grain pita bread, and as a sandwich spread.*

Basic Vinaigrette

Time: < 30 minutes   **Makes:** ¼ cup

- 1 tablespoon lemon juice or apple cider vinegar
- 3 tablespoons extra-virgin olive oil
- salt and pepper, to taste

Whisk the ingredients together until well combined. Use immediately or store in an airtight container in the refrigerator for up to 2 weeks. Freezing is not recommended.

Raspberry Vinaigrette

Time: < 30 minutes   **Makes:** about 1¼ cups

- 1 cup frozen raspberries
- ¼ cup balsamic vinegar
- ¼ cup red wine vinegar
- ½ cup extra-virgin olive oil
- 1 small shallot, minced
- 1 teaspoon Dijon mustard
- salt and pepper, to taste

In a blender, combine the raspberries, vinegars, oil, shallot, and mustard until smooth. Season to taste, and set aside for at least 10 minutes before serving for flavor development. Use immediately or store in an airtight container in the refrigerator for up to 1 week. Freezing is not recommended.

French Vinaigrette

Time: < 30 minutes   **Makes:** ½ to ⅔ cup

2 tablespoons minced shallots

2 tablespoons champagne vinegar

¼ teaspoon salt

2 teaspoons Dijon mustard

4–6 tablespoons extra-virgin olive oil

freshly ground pepper, to taste

Combine all the ingredients except the oil and pepper, then slowly whisk in the oil until the dressing reaches the desired consistency. Taste and season with pepper to taste. Use immediately or store in an airtight container in the refrigerator for up to 1 week. Freezing is not recommended.

Mediterranean Vinaigrette

Time: < 30 minutes   **Makes:** ¼ cup

1 tablespoon red wine vinegar

1 teaspoon pomegranate juice

3 tablespoons extra-virgin olive oil

½ clove garlic, minced

½ teaspoon dried oregano

salt and pepper, to taste

Whisk together all the ingredients until well combined, and season with salt and pepper to taste. Use immediately or store in an airtight container in the refrigerator for up to 1 week. Freezing is not recommended.

Honey Dijon Vinaigrette

Time: < 30 minutes   **Makes:** about ½ cup

3 tablespoons extra-virgin olive oil

zest and juice from 1 medium lemon

1 teaspoon Dijon mustard

1 clove garlic, minced

½ teaspoon grated ginger

¼ teaspoon honey

Whisk together all the ingredients until well combined. Use immediately or store in an airtight container in the refrigerator for up to 1 week. Freezing is not recommended.

Plant-Based Parmesan

Time: <30 minutes   **Makes:** about 1½ cups

1 cup raw cashews

¼ cup nutritional yeast

½ teaspoon garlic powder

½ teaspoon onion powder

¼ teaspoon salt

Place all the ingredients in a food processor and pulse to the desired crumb consistency, but before the mixture becomes creamy or liquefied. Use immediately or store in an airtight container in the refrigerator for up to 3 months, or freeze for up to 6 months.

Tip: *Use anywhere you'd use grated Parmesan—on pasta dishes, savory toast, eggs, and salads.*

Cashew Crema

Time: < 30 minutes plus soaking time   **Makes:** about 1¼ cups

1 cup raw cashews

6 tablespoons fresh lemon juice (about 2 lemons)

¼ teaspoon sea salt

1 teaspoon nutritional yeast

½ cup water or plain unsweetened almond milk

1. Soak the cashews 2 hours to overnight.

2. Using a high-powered blender, combine all the ingredients and blend until creamy, about 1 minute. Let cool completely. Use immediately or store in an airtight container in the refrigerator for up to 1 week, or freeze for up to 1 month.

Tip: Use this crema anywhere you'd use sour cream—in tacos, soups, herby dips, and creamy dressings.

CONVERSIONS

Common Conversions

1 gallon = 4 quarts = 8 pints = 16 cups = 128 fluid ounces = 3.8 liters
1 quart = 2 pints = 4 cups = 32 ounces = .95 liter
1 pint = 2 cups = 16 ounces = 480 ml
1 cup = 8 ounces = 240 ml
¼ cup = 4 tablespoons = 12 teaspoons = 2 ounces = 60 ml

Temperature Conversions

FAHRENHEIT (°F)	CELSIUS (°C)
200°F	95°C
225°F	110°C
250°F	120°C
275°F	135°C
300°F	150°C
325°F	165°C
350°F	175°C
375°F	190°C
400°F	200°C
425°F	220°C
450°F	230°C
475°F	245°C

Volume Conversions

U.S.	U.S. EQUIVALENT	METRIC
1 tablespoon (3 teaspoons)	½ fluid ounce	15 milliliters
¼ cup	2 fluid ounces	60 milliliters
⅓ cup	3 fluid ounces	80 milliliters
½ cup	4 fluid ounces	120 milliliters
⅔ cup	5 fluid ounces	160 milliliters
¾ cup	6 fluid ounces	180 milliliters
1 cup	8 fluid ounces	240 milliliters
2 cups	16 fluid ounces	480 milliliters

Weight Conversions

U.S.	METRIC
½ ounce	15 grams
1 ounce	30 grams
2 ounces	60 grams
¼ pound	115 grams
⅓ pound	150 grams
½ pound	225 grams
¾ pound	340 grams
1 pound	450 grams

RECIPE INDEX

ACKNOWLEDGMENTS

This book is dedicated to Fred, the one I want to grow old with. He's the reason I want as many healthy years on this Earth as possible—so we can continue our life of play and adventure without limitation. That is my wish for both of us, and for all of you.

My parents seem to be doing something right too. Pushing 80, and still out there running around. Maybe it's all that kimchi (probiotics!).

For support from afar, thanks go to my three sisters and brother, Ahrie, Gurie, Suerie, and Kahmyong, on whom I know I can depend though we occupy three continents between us.

Finally, thanks go to the team at Ulysses Press, especially my editor Casie Vogel, and the rest of the editors and designers that make my words look good.

ABOUT THE AUTHOR

Maggie Moon, MS, RD, is the best-selling author of *The MIND Diet* (Ulysses Press, 2016), and lead author of the "Medical Nutrition Therapy for Neurologic Disorders" textbook chapter in the 15th edition of *Krause's Food and Nutrition Care Process* (Elsevier, 2019). Her nutrition work has taken her across America and around the world: from NYC public schools to national commodity boards, from supermarket sustainable seafood programs to multi-billion-dollar global food companies. Ms. Moon's unique career has been profiled in *Today's Dietitian*, *Launching Your Dietetics Career*, and DiversifyDietetics.org, an online community that empowers students and young professionals from underrepresented minority groups to join the next generation of nutrition experts.

She completed her clinical training at New York Presbyterian Hospital of Columbia and Cornell, and holds a master of science degree in nutrition and education from Columbia University's Teachers College, with a bachelor of arts degree in English literature from U.C. Berkeley. Her culinary school training is from The New School of Cooking in Los Angeles, California. After a decade in New York City, she and her husband now live in Los Angeles, where they strive to spend more time eating amazing produce than sitting in traffic.